The
HOMEGROWN
HERBAL
APOTHECARY

120+ Easy-to-Grow Plants
for Healing Remedies

DEVON YOUNG

Author of
The Backyard Herbal Apothecary and
Creator of Nitty Gritty Life

Illustrated by Hanna Martin

PAGE STREET
PUBLISHING CO.

PAGE STREET
PUBLISHING CO.

Copyright © 2023 Devon Young

First published in 2023 by
Page Street Publishing Co.
27 Congress Street, Suite 1511
Salem, MA 01970
www.pagestreetpublishing.com

Distributed by Macmillan, sales in Canada by The Canadian Manda Group.

27 26 25 24 23   1 2 3 4 5

ISBN-13: 978-1-64567-864-9
ISBN-10: 1-64567-864-4

Library of Congress Control Number: 2023936668

Cover and book design by Vienna Mercedes Gambol for Page Street Publishing Co.
Illustrations by Hanna Martin
Plant Hardiness Zone Map on page 17 from the U.S. Department of Agriculture
Agricultural Research Service

Printed and bound in China

This book is dedicated to all those who have endured and
supported my love of plants, but particularly to my grandparents,
Darrell and Betty, for showing me that a life with a little dirt
under your nails is a life well lived.

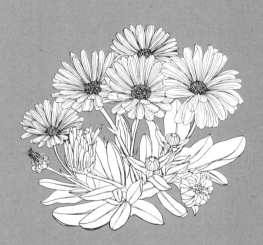

CONTENTS

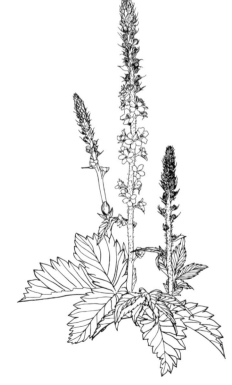

Introduction

Gardening is among the very earliest memories in my life.

My fascination with and appreciation for the botanical world when I was young. It seems we always had a garden, no matter how big or small—there was always a vegetable patch each summer that I would help tend to with my parents. My maternal grandparents had a sizable acreage and a garden that wrapped three sides of their substantial yard, always filled with sunny marigolds, just beyond the fruit tree border, before the land stretched into the pastures beyond. I spent endless summers planting, weeding, watering and harvesting these crops and more yet, enjoying the beautiful flower gardens that my grandmother lovingly arranged. Tucked up on a rock wall, in the shade of the cherry tree, amongst the snapdragons or swinging from the swing suspended from the majestic oaks, I was a kid at peace.

My love of the plant kingdom never really ebbed as I aged into my teenage years. I found myself asking for seed packets, soil and trays to plant herbs in each spring for my April birthday. I found myself growing to understand that culinary herbs, pretty flowers and various plants that surrounded us had use beyond flavor and ornamentation. I spent countless hours at the library, seeking and checking out books on herbs, piling far more into my backpack than was comfortable.

As a young adult, and eventually as a mother, I sought out ways to nourish and heal my family. I grew my own gardens and raised my own food. I started dipping my toes into home remedies. I learned that I didn't have to opt in fully to the modern, conventional, consumer-driven and allopathic model. I found that a convenient, paint-by-numbers lifestyle didn't sit well with me (though I am not shaming those who choose this direction out of necessity or lack of knowledge and skill). I was simply more comfortable and fulfilled in caring for my loved ones myself.

I became an herbalist.

My path into herbalism meandered as I learned. Like any eager student, the allure of exotic and rare herbs had a great appeal, but I knew fundamentally that healing and health could be achieved close to the literal and metaphorical home. The notion that perhaps we have mostly everything we need to thrive near us, if we only knew what to look for and how to care for and prepare it, became a driving focus in my practice and lifestyle. My blog Nitty Gritty Life was born, where I have explored topics relating to holistic and sustainable living.

But even within the complementary and alternative medicine world, I found that there was a very large, even oppressive component of consumerism—wellness products, wellness services, wellness as a BRAND. I observed so many companies promoting natural healing in a very "this for that" allopathic model. Like so many herbalists before me, this notion felt like it flew in the face of herbalism. At the core, herbalism is finding balance and synergy with the natural world while achieving a healthy neutral within us. And it is in this concept that I have worked to educate myself and others in how to take a proactive approach to healing at home.

Growing the herbs that we use to remedy our complaints feels like such a natural component of herbalism. It respects nature, lowers our footprint and lessens our impact on the environment. With these thoughts in mind, the concept of this book was born. The very soil surrounding our homes could very well provide much of the nourishment and healing that we need to thrive. We can turn our landscapes—as small as a balcony terrace or as large as a sprawling acreage—into a healing oasis. Furthermore, these healing gardens can be beautiful as well as functional.

We can grow health and wellness at home.

My goal with this book is to teach you that there is little separation between the garden and the apothecary and that there can be fluid, uninterrupted motion from seed and root to remedy and health. I want you to think like an herbalist in the garden and think like a gardener in the apothecary. In doing so, we can achieve a degree of sustainability and, dare I say, self-sufficiency. We can regard the very land we live on as the fundamental building block for our health and vitality.

I want to foster you with a sense of empowerment and confidence that is supported by knowledge, so that you can begin to think, "I know this, I got this, I can do this" and not slip into the analysis paralysis that so many of us do when confronted with the wide breadth of herbalism.

In this book, you will find the first chapters devoted to understanding your garden's potential and some of the core concepts of home herbalism. We will explore straightforward topics such as soil, climate, growing zones and why those are important to the health and potency of healing botanicals, while also dipping our toes into more esoteric concepts of moon cycle gardening and creating unique healing spaces within the landscape. We will also take a moment to simplify the complexity of herbalism and lean into our own inherent intuition and learned knowledge to create healing remedies from the herbs we grow. Using basic remedy formulations for teas, tinctures, infusions and more, we can use these preparations for each herb in this book and the thousands of others that I simply could not conceive of covering in one set of pages.

The herbal profiles are our "snapshots" into the medicinal benefits of each botanical, how to grow it in our landscapes, when to harvest it and how to use each herb. These profiles are designed to be a launching point for home herbalists and gardeners alike to dive into the deep end of these amazing medicinal allies. These profiles are intended to help you see your landscape through a new lens. In the latter part of this book, you will find a therapeutic action index for each herb mentioned to encourage independent study of these botanicals and how to best utilize their health and wellness benefits.

I hope you find this book to be a useful guide and resource to cultivating a medicinal landscape. I hope that the topics discussed will encourage both herbalists and gardeners to create their gardens and apothecaries with a sense of independence and "can do" spirit. I hope you will grow as both a gardener and home herbalist.

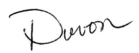

Understanding Herbal Energetics & The Doctrine of Signatures

When I became acquainted with the concept of herbal energetics, it was like the door burst open on the vast world of herbal knowledge. No longer did I feel like I needed to memorize the therapeutic actions and medicinal uses of hundreds or even thousands of herbs. Instead, I just needed to know the core basics of herbs as they related to us.

Herbal energetics are explained somewhat differently within the various cultural healing modalities such as Traditional Chinese Medicine, Ayurveda and Western herbalism. While these different models may appear separate at face value, they all seek to achieve the same ends—to relieve exaggerated conditions and return the mind and body back to a healthy neutrality.

I practice a Western approach to herbalism. In Western herbalism, conditions and our core constitutions, as well as the herbal remedies that we use are classified as warm or cool and dry or damp. It seems impossibly simple, but reducing complexities to simple terms can be incredibly insightful. Our energetic state may be constitutional; i.e., our basic everyday tendency in a relatively healthy state, or altered or exacerbated by conditions such as illness or injury. As herbalists, we seek to bring individuals as close to a healthy neutral as possible by choosing herbs that offset exaggerated states. In Western herbalism, we classify people, health complaints and herbs in the following ways: warm/dry, warm/damp, cool/dry and cool/damp.

WARM

Warm people exhibit, obviously, warmth. This may be a very literal warmth—the type of human space heaters that radiate heat. More complex than simple temperature, warm people tend to have a natural flush about their skin, which may even present as a red or ruddy complexion, red mucous membrane, noticeable capillaries in the eyes and a red tongue, indented with teeth imprints. A warm person's demeanor may be inviting and bold, but may also be given to anger and agitation.

Warm conditions are often related to acute infection and traumatic injury but may also be indicative of a bodily system that is working too hard to maintain itself. These are conditions of over-excitement and over-compensation.

Warm herbs are typically stimulating and diffusive in nature. They are often aromatic, spicy, and pungent. We use warming herbs to negate cold, depressed, "stuck" conditions like sinus pressure, stiff joints and poor circulation. Examples of warm herbs include:

- *Cayenne (page 122)*
- *Bee Balm (page 63)*
- *Oregano (page 112)*
- *Thyme (page 105)*
- *Angelica (page 37)*

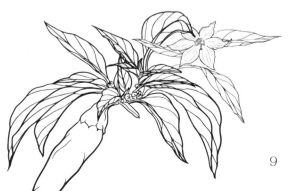

COOL

Cool folks are quite often cold to the touch, like their baseline temperature runs at the lower end of the thermometer. It is as if their visceral internal heat doesn't quite radiate to the distal ends of their extremities. Cool people often have a bluer tone to their skin, pale pink mucous membranes, white clear eyes and a tongue that presents with a white or gray cast. The personality of a cool person may appear dreamier and more carefree, even distant and aloof at times.

Cool conditions are often a sign of chronic illness or disease, or diminished organ function. These are conditions of exhaustion and debility.

Cool herbs tend to be calming and reductive in nature. Aromatic herbs thought of as cooling usually land on the mintier, floral/fruity and earthy end of the scent spectrum, while many don't have pronounced scents at all. Cooling herbs relieve heightened conditions such as fever, swollen and arthritic joints and sensations of extreme visceral heat. Example of cool herbs include:

— *Lemon Balm (page 55)*

— *Catmint (page 31)*

— *Sage (page 35)*

— *Mugwort (page 128)*

— *Stinging Nettle (page 140)*

DRY

Dry individuals quite often have dehydrated skin, prone to ashiness and flaking. They may blink often, have pronounced texture to the fingerprints, a tendency to be itchy, hair that may appear dull and their tongue may appear cracked or have a sandpaper-like texture. Dry individuals are often serious in nature and have a tendency to be deep thinkers, prone to contemplation.

Dry conditions present themselves when the body is in an undernourished/dehydrated state, be that from an actual lack of nourishment or the lack of ability to utilize nourishment in food or from dehydration due to lack of fluid intake or disproportionate fluid output (think sweating, vomiting or diarrhea). A dry condition demonstrates that the body is unable to lubricate itself well.

Dry herbs staunch the flow of fluids from busted capillaries (think bruises), broken or effusive skin and leaky mucous membranes. Dry herbs may be leafy, but we often see inner barks and sometimes roots in this category. Examples of dry herbs include:

— *Tea (black or green) (page 22)*

— *Oregon Grape (page 81)*

— *Wormwood (page 103)*

— *Pine (page 116)*

— *Raspberry (leaf) (page 62)*

DAMP

Damp persons often have shiny skin that may feel either greasy (hot folks) or clammy (cold people) to the touch. Their eyes and hair may appear shiny, their mucous membranes are glossy and their tongues are often noticeably wet. A damp persona is often outgoing and talkative, even generous in nature.

Damp conditions are suggestive of damaged tissues and imbalanced and overactive organs. It is a condition of excess often observed in the common cold and diarrhea.

Damp herbs are moist and often highly nutritive. These herbs are often from fruits, flowers, leaves and sometimes roots.

Examples of damp herbs include:

- *Marshmallow (page 127)*
- *Calendula (page 73)*
- *Licorice (page 126)*
- *Violet (page 95)*
- *Aloe (page 114)*

With an understanding of energetics, we can pair individuals with herbs that will best remedy their complaints. We can dial down heat, or raise the temperature, we can flood a human desert or staunch the flood of fluids by choosing an "opposing" herb to counteract a condition or state. We can return the mind and body to a stasis, a state of neutral adaptability. We can restore health and wellness.

DOCTRINE OF SIGNATURES

One almost intangible concept in herbalism is the doctrine of signatures. This is the notion that the physical characteristics, growth habits, preferred habitat and other features of a botanical are suggestive of its medicinal use. Perhaps this is how medicine people for thousands of years, before modern science, came to experiment with plants to remedy maladies of the mind and body. Early healers used their intuition to guide their choices when selecting plants for medicine making.

Modern herbalists can apply the doctrine of signatures as a springboard to great herbal knowledge. When observing a botanical, what features stand out? What images does it conjure? How does it make one feel in its presence?

Here are a few questions to ask when in the presence of a potential healing ally:

- Does part of the plant resemble human anatomy? Example: mullein flowers resemble ears.

- What colors are presenting themselves in the fruit, flowers, bark, pithy wood and roots? Color is often indicative of health benefits. Examples: yellow often suggests antimicrobial action, red/purple may support cardiovascular health.

- How do the tissues, such as stalk or stem, respond to movement? Are they rigid and firm, or yielding and flexible? Think about how a sunflower follows the sun and how that may promote flexibility and mobility.

- Do the aromatics transport your spirit? Does lavender offer you relaxation, does a rose awaken a sense of sensuality?

- What do various structures of the plant say? Think about the downy, absorptive leaves of lamb's ear or the deep mineral sequestering taproots of wild carrot.

- Is the plant soft and welcoming or thorny and formidable? Consider the less scientific aspects of the thorns of hawthorn helping one to establish personal boundaries.

- How does the plant feel between your fingers? Imagine the sting of nettle bringing healthy, oxygen-rich blood to the skin surface or the resinous exudate of calendula soothing and sealing a wound.

So much can be learned through thoughtful observation, and I invite you all on an herbal learning journey to sit with a plant and simply take in its presence with all your senses.

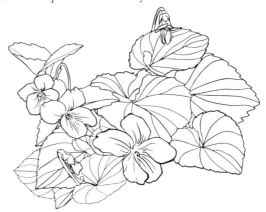

The Simple Science & Magic of Growing

Growing plants offers a satisfying abundance and sense of accomplishment when one is successful in their endeavors. But in order to reap the bounty of a successful healing garden, it is important to understand the basics of soil, fertility and natural cycles that create the magic that is growing.

Gardening is an act of adapting to our surroundings. Weather, soil conditions and even the placement of buildings, fences and trees may dictate, to some degree, the plants that will grow in a certain landscape. It is not particularly wise to force our will upon natural spaces as it rarely ends in success. But when we work in tandem with Mother Nature, we can achieve the goal of vitality in the garden and wellness from the apothecary. We can create garden spaces perfectly suited to our settings full of healing herbs.

In this chapter, you will learn the basic foundational tenets of gardening and how that translates to choosing the herbs best suited to your landscape—be that a shady balcony of containers or a sprawling acreage in full sun. By understanding the unique conditions and requirements for your garden, you can then select for success, rather than forcing plants to exist in conditions that may not be suitable for their vitality.

SOIL

At a local and regional level, soil science can seem incredibly complex, layered and nuanced. The soil in a given area develops and evolves from ecological occurrences, wildlife grazing, livestock management and manmade construction developments. These things shape and shift the soil into what we see and call "dirt."

One can certainly dive deep to learn about their specific location's unique soil structure utilizing the knowledge of scientists, university records, municipal and governmental resources and the experience of neighboring farmers and gardeners.

But for the purposes of this book, that's not necessary. Experiencing the soil with all of your senses, especially touch, sight and even smell, and learning the basic soil vocabulary that you will see in this book and elsewhere, will turn a novice gardener into an expert of their own backyard.

We can, of course, aggressively amend soils with "off-farm" inputs purchased from big box stores and garden supply centers. This may help us to rebuild a healthy soil system, but more often than not, it is a self-perpetuating cycle of buying MORE—hardly economical, ecological or sustainable. While I am certainly not averse to amending as needed, or for the creation of raised beds, the more holistic approach I recommend for your medicinal garden journey is to select plants that are naturally suited to your home soil condition.

I invite you to grab a shovel and dig into several areas of your landscape. How does the soil appear? What does it feel like? Does it have a distinctive aroma? Below, I have described each soil type, the unique identifiers to look for and how to make the best of them. These are listed from the heaviest and densest to the lightest and most permeable soil types.

Clay

Clay soils are dense and heavy, with fine particles that pack closely together. This soil will hold its shape when formed or molded while wet. These soils are often fertile, but due to the tight structure of the soil, nutrient availability may be poor. These soils retain excessive moisture and can become boggy and swamp-like during heavy precipitation, while also becoming rock hard and bone-dry during times of drought. These soils are often found in flood plains, notably in areas of human development such as neighborhoods and cities, and near roadways due to the compacting nature of construction and development.

When selecting medicinal herbs for heavy clay soils, consider plants with deep, soil mining taproots and extensive, even aggressive root systems. Think of cultivars of wild plants that we observe growing roadside, in neglected spaces, and those that thrive in high traffic areas. These types of plants are well suited to heavy, dense soils. A small sampling of plants that thrive in clay soils includes:

- *St. John's Wort (page 56)*
- *Queen Anne's Lace/Wild Carrot (page 47)*
- *Chicory (page 45)*
- *Mullein (page 34)*
- *Oregon Grape (page 81)*

Silty

Silty soils have a slippery, flour-like feel and are fine textured. The particles will hold together when formed but with less density and firmness than clay. During types of heavy precipitation, silt can become boggy and it is prone to erosion. This soil type tends to be moderately rich in fertility. Silty soils are formed by river, lake and pond edges.

When confronted with siltier soils, a gardener should consider those plants that naturally thrive near fresh waterways such as rivers, ponds, creeks and lakes. Some plants that sit well in silt include:

- *Cottonwood (page 121)*
- *Birch (page 119)*
- *Meadowsweet (page 77)*
- *Milkweed/Pleurisy Root (page 66)*
- *Gravel Root (Joe Pye Weed) (page 132)*

Loam

This soil structure is considered ideal for most garden conditions. It is a balanced blend of particles that allow roots to move freely underground with high nutrient value and will only loosely hold together if formed while wet. Loamy soils drain freely even in heavy precipitation but retain moisture well. Loamy soils are often found in naturalized areas (those undeveloped areas abundant in native vegetation) such as prairies and grasslands, valleys and agricultural areas. If there is a lush and thriving farming community nearby, chances are your soil resembles a fertile loam.

Being a fairly ideal soil structure, common medicinal and edibles are particularly fond of this type of dirt. Here is where just about anything will thrive. A sampling of loam-loving plants include:

- *Cayenne (page 122)*
- *Calendula (page 73)*
- *Mint (page 41)*
- *Dill (page 38)*
- *Cornsilk (page 46)*

Humus

These types of soils are abundant in decayed plant and animal matter, and the particles are rarely very uniform in structure due to the diverse organic material. They are often dark in color, highly aromatic, moisture-retentive and very fertile. Humus rich soils are often found in forests, woodlands, open meadows and areas of very diverse plant material and wildlife and very little human interruption.

Think of the forest floor when selecting herbs for humus-y soils. These herbs play well in a diverse landscape and tend to not be overly competitive for resources. Some humus happy plants include:

- *Violet (page 95)*
- *Wild Ginger (page 125)*
- *Stinging Nettle (page 140)*
- *Lungwort (page 148)*
- *Cottonwood (page 121)*

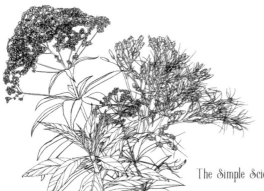

Sandy

Sandy soils are porous, composed of large particles and loose in structure. These soils tend to be of very poor fertility and create some of the harsher conditions for a plant to grow in. Sandy soils have very poor water retention and will not hold together well when formed while wet. Sandy soils are found in arid regions and along coastlines.

Where there are sandy soils present, seek out hardy plants with somewhat shallow root systems and a slightly waxy coating to the foliage. These adaptations prevent moisture loss and ensure the longevity of the plants. Plants that tolerate sandy soils include:

—— *Lavender (page 110)*

—— *Aloe (page 114)*

—— *Rosemary (page 100)*

—— *Sea Buckthorn (page 104)*

—— *Juniper (page 99)*

FERTILITY

Soil fertility is defined by the elements of the soil. While many elements are important to the health and vigor of plant life, there are three elements that are fundamental to all botanicals. These are nitrogen, potassium and phosphorus. These fundamental nutrients nourish specific times in a plant's growth cycle and support the health and integrity of a plant's "anatomy." This is of particular importance when we consider the parts of plants we use as herbalists. Nitrogen, phosphorus and potassium availability will help ensure that the leaves, flowers, fruits, roots and stems that we harvest have the maximum healing potential.

While not entirely necessary for the home herbal gardener, soil testing can provide insight to the nutrient availability of one's land. Simple soil testing kits are readily available online and in farm and garden stores, while more extensive testing can be done at universities and laboratories that can provide additional insight. Once an herbal gardener has a gauge on their soil nutrient profile,

they may choose whether to amend the soil with fertilizers (which may be necessary if the nutrient availability of a soil is particularly poor) or adjust your plant selection according to your native soil conditions to ensure success.

Nitrogen (N): Nitrogen is considered perhaps the most important element for plants. This element is essential to the formation of the protein necessary to build cells and allow growth. Nitrogen is essential for the formation of chlorophyll and promotes photosynthesis. Nitrogen deficient plants appear yellowed and dull.

Plentiful nitrogen will be a requirement for gardeners that want densely planted lush gardens with extensive foliage and vegetative growth. Nitrogen-rich soils are excellent for traditionally heavy feeders, such as corn and many traditionally cultivated foliage dense plants, and those with somewhat shallow root systems. Consider the primary plant parts used when selecting for nitrogen-rich soils—those where leaves are the great medicinal value will likely need nitrogen-rich soils. Examples of plants that enjoy abundant nitrogen include:

—— *Sage (page 35)*

—— *Mint (page 41)*

—— *Lemon balm (page 55)*

—— *Artichoke (page 48)*

—— *Cornsilk (page 46)*

When deficiency of nitrogen is present in the native soil, consider less "leafy" plants that are more succulent or evergreen in nature. Some healing herbs that will do well in nitrogen-deficient conditions are:

—— *Aloe (page 114)*

—— *Yucca (page 98)*

—— *Pine (page 116)*

—— *Juniper (page 99)*

—— *Sea Buckthorn (page 104)*

Phosphorus (P): Phosphorus is necessary for the development of a healthy root system and facilitates the energy transfer between the different types of tissues in plants and the flowering and fruiting process. Phosphorus deficient plants may appear puny and lack vigor and have greatly diminished flowering and fruiting capacity. Additionally, leaves may appear mottled and not uniformly green.

Phosphorus helps facilitate those herbs whose root, flowers and fruits will be used. These medicinals are best suited to phosphorus-abundant soils:

- *Passionflower (page 86)*
- *Cranberry (page 131)*
- *Calendula (page 73)*
- *Valerian (page 138)*
- *Marshmallow (page 127)*

Where phosphorus is less plentiful, consider botanicals that don't produce fruits and that are not particularly "floral" and somewhat compact in form, such as:

- *Mugwort (page 128)*
- *Mullein (page 34)*
- *Wormwood (page 103)*
- *Wild Ginger (page 125)*

Potassium (K): Potassium provides the nutrients needed for vigor and stress adaptability, while also promoting the flowering and fruiting cycles. Plants deficient in potassium will have a reduced rate of photosynthesis and tissues will appear damaged, withered, wilted, browned and mushy.

Potassium content is key for those herbs grown in a high potential stress environment, particularly those in arid, drought-prone areas. Herbs that enjoy the benefit of ample potassium include:

- *Peach (page 42)*
- *Pumpkin (page 60)*
- *Oregon Grape (page 81)*
- *Calendula (page 73)*

Some succulent and evergreen botanicals can flourish in spite of somewhat potassium-deficient soils. These include:

- *Aloe (page 114)*
- *Pine (page 116)*
- *Juniper (page 99)*
- *Rosemary (page 100)*
- *Sage (page 35)*

pH

Soil pH measures the respective acidity versus alkalinity present. Measured on a scale of 0 to 14, with 7 considered neutral, acidic conditions exist below a measure of seven (low pH) and alkaline conditions exist above seven (high pH). Home gardeners can measure the pH of their soils with inexpensive testing kits readily available online and in farm and garden stores. Most plants thrive in neutral to slightly acidic conditions between 6.5 and 7.0 pH because this is the pH in which phosphorus, as well as many other nutrients, is most soluble. It is usually unnecessary to amend or alter the soil pH if your native soil falls in the range of 6.5 and 7.5. However, certain plants have preference or requirement for certain pH conditions, while others will alter their form or color in response to the acidity or alkalinity.

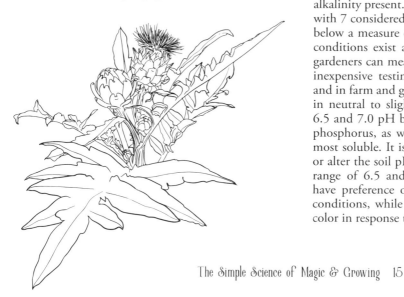

Acidity: Acidic soil conditions occur where there is accumulation of diverse, decaying plant matter. The conditions are also associated with regions of great rainfall, or even extreme irrigation or controlled flooding as a high volume of water will leach alkaline components such as calcium, magnesium and potassium from the soil. Excessive use of nitrogen fertilizer will also decrease soil pH.

Your soil might be slightly acidic to very acidic if you find that grass in your lawn is patchy, sparse and prone to moss. Foliage may yellow or brown prematurely. Plants that thrive in relatively acidic soil conditions include:

- *Pine (page 116)*
- *Oak (page 70)*
- *Fir (page 146)*
- *Camellia (page 78)*

Alkalinity: Alkaline soils tend to be chalky and porous and comparatively low in organic matter, while being high in calcium, magnesium and sodium. These high pH conditions are often present in arid areas with low annual rainfall. High alkalinity soils can also be caused by excessive lime application.

Signs that your soil may be highly alkaline are curled and wilted leaves, purplish stems and a general dehydrated, droopy appearance. However, some plants that will tolerate more alkaline soils conditions include:

- *California Poppy (page 51)*
- *Red Clover (page 61)*
- *Borage (page 30)*
- *Lavender (page 110)*
- *Crampbark (page 142)*

SUN EXPOSURE

Plants require sunlight to photosynthesize but to varying degrees. Some botanicals thrive in full, radiant sun, others enjoy deep shade, while many others enjoy the liminal space between. Each herb profiled in this book will have suggested sun exposure requirements. Choose your plants and their placement based in their lighting needs to avoid underwhelming performance and set your healing garden up for success.

Full Sun: Plants that prefer full sun require at least 6 hours of unfiltered sun exposure per day.

Partial Shade: Partial-shade plants thrive in 3 to 6 hours of direct exposure. These plants often do better when sheltered from harsh late afternoon rays.

Full Shade: Full-shade plants require less than 3 hours of sun exposure. Some of these plants prefer dappled light under an open canopy of trees, while still others enjoy the deeper darkness of a forest.

GROWING ZONES

For the purposes of this book, I will be referencing the USDA's designated growing zones. These are regional zones designated by average low temperatures. This is particularly important when choosing plants for your landscape. Using growing zone designations, gardeners can choose botanicals that are hardy in that climate or region.

Hardiness refers to a plant's ability to return each growing season and survive the low temperatures observed during the winter months. Perennial plants return year after year in their preferred growing zones. Some plants are considered "short-lived perennials" that typically only live for a few growing seasons in a given zone before losing vigor—often spreading by seed, rhizome or "suckers" before the mother plant dies. Annuals are plants that will typically die after one growing season, either as a function of the natural life cycle of the plant (grows for one season and reseeds) or because the botanical is actually perennial but grown outside its preferred growing zone. For instance, we see this with more tropical plants grown in cooler, temperate climates.

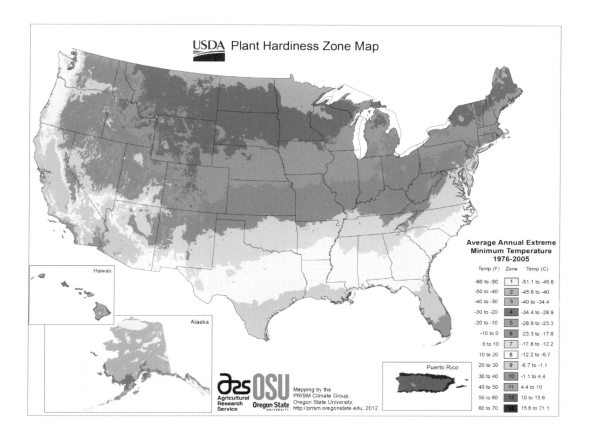

USDA Plant Hardiness Zone Map

Average Annual Extreme Minimum Temperature 1976-2005

Temp (F)	Zone	Temp (C)
-60 to -50	1	-51.1 to -45.6
-50 to -40	2	-45.6 to -40
-40 to -30	3	-40 to -34.4
-30 to -20	4	-34.4 to -28.9
-20 to -10	5	-28.9 to -23.3
-10 to 0	6	-23.3 to -17.8
0 to 10	7	-17.8 to -12.2
10 to 20	8	-12.2 to -6.7
20 to 30	9	-6.7 to -1.1
30 to 40	10	-1.1 to 4.4
40 to 50	11	4.4 to 10
50 to 60	12	10 to 15.6
60 to 70	13	15.6 to 21.1

Mapping by the PRISM Climate Group, Oregon State University. http://prism.oregonstate.edu, 2012

Agricultural Research Service OSU Oregon State University

SEED SOWING

Once a botanical has been selected for growing, one of the most economical ways to enjoy this plant is by growing it from seed. While I have outlined basic seed-sowing guidelines in the plant profiles, individual selections may have more specific requirements. Always read your seed packets carefully to ensure success with specific varieties and cultivars. Here are some questions to ask yourself as you prepare to plant seeds:

Does this seed prefer to be covered with soil and if so, how deep should it be planted?

Does this seed need light to germinate, meaning that it should only be in firm contact with the soil surface?

What temperature range is suggested for germination?

How moist should the starting medium be kept?

Are there specific requirements of the soil medium itself?

Does this seed require scarification, meaning the surface of the seed needs to be nicked or abraded?

Should this seed be soaked prior to planting?

What is the anticipated germination window?

———— Does this seed require cold stratification (a period of cold exposure that can be achieved by sowing directly in the desired location in fall to overwinter, or in early spring while the weather is still moist and cold, or by chilling moistened seeds in the refrigerator)?

SEED SAVING

One of the ultimate acts of sustainability is seed saving. Here are some helpful hints when it comes to collecting seeds from your healing garden bounty.

———— Most seeds need to reach full maturity while still on the plant in order to be viable.

———— While some seeds like calendula are easily collected from the spent flower head, others, especially those with tiny seeds, require some protection while they are being collected. Secure a small paper bag or seed envelope around the seed's head when fully mature and dry to the touch. Cut the plant's stem and shake or dislodge the seeds with your fingers into the bag or envelope.

———— Seeds and nuts collected from nut trees (such as black walnut) and fruiting trees and plants will often require a period of rotting away the fleshy outer coating, then drying of the seeds to save for future planting.

———— Remove all foreign matter and make sure the seeds are completely dry before storage. Store seeds for 1 to 2 years (although some seeds remain viable longer), in a cool, dry dark place.

———— Sow older seeds more thickly as seed viability tends to diminish over time.

———— Some varieties of plants, like roses and certain types of lavender, are hybridized, meaning that the "parent material" for that plant are from different species within that genus. As such, seeds from these plants may not produce a new generation with the same characteristics.

MOON CYCLE GARDENING

Most of us who live along coastlines have observed the higher tides experienced during a full moon, and conversely lower tides observed during a new moon. This phenomenon is due to the gravitational pull of the moon. This phenomenon extends beyond the ocean to the plant kingdom. Gardeners can apply this knowledge to our planting, harvesting and even fertilizing schedules.

This concept can be explored in much greater depth but is most simply applied as follows:

Ascending or Waxing to Full Moon: This is a time of increasing lunar pull, bringing fluids UP. As such, this is an ideal time to sow seeds. As moisture seeps into the walls of a seed, the water promotes germination and sprouting transpires. This is also the best time to harvest aerial parts of botanicals, as the water and nutrients are drawn upward into the plant, increasing its constituent profile.

Descending or Waning to New Moon: During this time, the lunar pull decreases and fluids and nutrients are at a greater abundance to the roots of a plant. This is an ideal time to transplant seedlings as the decreased lunar pull will cause roots to seek a deeper home in the soil. It is also a good time to apply compost, as liquid, granular or foliar fertilizers and amendments. Additionally, this is a great time to harvest roots.

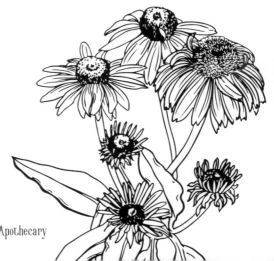

Creating Healing Garden Vignettes

Planting a beautiful healing garden takes special consideration of each plant's specific needs and the specific conditions present in your landscape and regions. Special care must be taken to group plants of similar requirements that will form a cohesive arrangement. While not all herbs with specific therapeutic actions are well suited to grow together, many are! When this stroke of serendipity occurs, we can cultivate these herbs together in healing vignettes or "mini gardens." These vignettes serve as a medicinal "garden tour" and offer the apothecary some targeted, strategized resources!

Once an herbalism-minded gardener has familiarized themselves with their specific soil, environmental and growing zone, they can then get to the good part: PLANTING!

While one can most certainly plant with no set plan, it can be logical, beautiful and fun to plant herbs with specific intention and actions in mind. Use the following suggestions as launching points to develop your own healing garden vignettes with plants of similar growing condition requirements.

THE SPICY DIFFUSIVE GARDEN

These herbs get things moving—breathing up congestion and stagnation. The tall spikes of garlic offset the lush foliage of oregano and bee balm, while diminutive thyme invites.

— *Garlic (page 36)*

— *Bee Balm (page 63)*

— *Oregano (page 112)*

— *Thyme (page 105)*

THE SOOTHING SPOT

Antispasmodic herbs and those that release anxiety and tension go hand in hand. Dill provides a tall backdrop to a wash of dreamy blues and purples provided by lavender and catmint, while sunny California poppy and chamomile bring bright charm and glow.

— *Lavender (page 110)*

— *Dill (page 38)*

— *Chamomile (German) (page 52)*

— *California Poppy (page 51)*

— *Catmint (page 31)*

CUT & COME AGAIN CULINARY CONTAINER

Equally culinary and medicinal, these plants are best grown close to the kitchen so one can impart their flavor and healing potential into everyday foods. Never forget that our health depends on the foods that we consume, so adding these flavorful and potent herbs to the diet makes for the best of both worlds.

— *Holy Basil/Tulsi (page 53)*

— *Sage (page 35)*

— *Rosemary (page 100)*

— *Mint (page 41) (Note: Grow mint in its own pot so it doesn't outcompete its neighbors)*

— *Coriander (page 49)*

— *Lovage (page 133)*

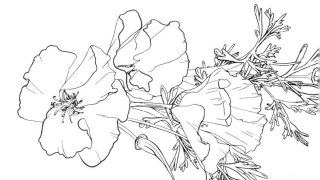

BREATHE EASY SPACE

Cool off and take a deep, lung-filling breath when surrounded by allies that promote respiratory wellness and ease coughs and sore throats. The staggering fir offers shade to the woodland herbs below.

- Fir (page 146)
- Oregon Grape (page 81)
- Meadowsweet (page 77)
- Violet (page 95)
- Wild Ginger (page 125)

MINDFULNESS RETREAT

Improve your clarity and focus while enjoying the beautiful array of these herbs, which promote brain power and that shine with shades of green, blue, purple and yellow.

- Rosemary (page 100)
- Holy Basil/Tulsi (page 53)
- Ashwagandha (page 50)
- St. John's Wort (page 56)

FIRST AID ALLIES

This grouping of profound wound healers can coexist in a dry, sunny garden to meet all your sudden needs for minor cuts, scrapes, sprains and strains.

- Calendula (page 73)
- Aloe (page 114)
- Yarrow (page 117)
- Arnica (page 72)

HEART'S EASE

Protect your heart and heal from trauma with these lovely, nurturing allies. These soft and gentle herbs will deliver the mind and heart to a place of healing and rest.

- Hawthorn (page 124)
- Mimosa (page 136)
- Vervain (page 139)
- Bacopa (page 134)
- Passionflower (page 86)

EVE'S GARDEN

This vignette is dedicated to the unique needs of a woman throughout her life. These are herbs to ease menstrual complaints and soothe the menopausal transition.

- Lady's Mantle (page 143)
- Black Cohosh (page 141)
- Motherwort (page 90)
- Mugwort (page 128)
- Crampbark (page 142)

IN THE FLOW

Here is an alliance of plants to release excessive fluids in the body and relieve a sense of being stuck and stagnant.

- Gravel Root (Joe Pye Weed)(page 132)
- Stinging Nettle (page 140)
- Hydrangea (page 84)

IMMUNITY OASIS

These are the herbs that will protect us from infectious illness, draw down a fever and promote well-being.

- Echinacea (page 44)
- Sea Buckthorn (page 104)
- Pine (page 116)
- Feverfew (page 33)
- Mint (page 41)

Preserving the Herbal Harvest & Stocking the Apothecary

DRYING FRESH HERBS FOR MEDICINE

Once the medicinal landscape has yielded an abundant harvest, the herbs must be preserved or crafted into remedies immediately. Before drying herbs for long-term preservation, herbs should be clean and free of debris, insects and potential chemical, fertilizer, road dust and animal urine/excrement contamination. Here are a few helpful guidelines for drying herbs for future use, depending on the type of plant matter.

Leaves: Leaves are perhaps the most abundant plant material at an herbalist's disposal. As such, we are often faced with abundance when it comes to drying this type of plant tissue. Traditionally, herbs are bundled and hung upside down, away from direct light. While this method is effective and aesthetically pleasing, leaves can be arranged in a single layer and dried at temperatures between 95 and 115°F (35 to 46°C).

Flowers: Several factors are involved in drying delicate flowers to preserve their aromatics and prevent browning. While small flowers such as chamomile can be dried intact, large, dense flowers such as certain roses should be de-petalled. Flowers and petals should be laid in a single layer and dried at temperatures no higher than 120°F (49°C).

Fruit: Due to the fleshy nature, special care must be taken to ensure that fruits do not mold or rot before they are adequately dry. While small berries like elderberry and vitex may dry quickly at dehydrator temperatures between 130 and 140°F (54 to 60°C), large fruits such as rosehips may dry better when halved before preserving.

Bark, Limbs and Roots: Due to the hard, supportive nature of roots, limbs and bark, this type of plant material should be trimmed or crumbled to its desired size before preservation.

This type of plant material should be laid out in a single layer and dried at temperatures ranging from 135 to 150°F (57 to 65°C).

Unopened Buds and Highly Resinous Material: Certain plant material such as cotton buds present a challenge in drying effectively. Due to density and resinous constituents, this type of plant material should be dried at temperatures ranging from 150 to 180°F (65 to 82°C). This material should feel almost brittle to the touch once cooled.

Once herbs are dried, they should be stored in an airtight container, in a cool location, away from direct light. Leafy and flower materials are typically most medicinally potent within approximately 4 years; bark, roots, limbs and properly preserved resinous buds may be vital for 2 years.

FREEZING FRESH HERBS FOR MEDICINE

This preservation method is so under-utilized in herbalism!

Freezing herbs is ideal for those types of herbs that don't dry easily due to mass or water content. It is also excellent for fruits and flowers where preservation of flavor, aroma and texture is desired.

Leaves and Flowers: This type of plant matter works best if finely chopped and placed in ice cube trays. Fill trays with water (or oil, such as olive oil, if desired) and freeze. Remove the cubes from the trays and place the cubes in an airtight container or freezer bag. Use within 1 year. Use herbal ice cubes crafted from aromatic herbs to flavor your favorite beverages, such as iced tea or sparkling water. Ice cubes with nutritive herbs like nettle can be stirred into soups or even blended into pestos and sauces. These herbal ice cubes may also be useful in various hot or cold infusions and decoctions.

Fruit and Buds: This type of plant matter is ideally frozen in a single layer on a rimmed baking sheet and transferred to a container or freezer bag when fully frozen. Alternatively, tiny fruits, such as elderberries, can be frozen still on the cluster/stems and then removed from the stems for long-term storage. Use these within 1 year. Fruits and buds preserved by freezing are perfect for syrups and honey fermentations or infusions.

Roots: This type of plant matter should be finely chopped or shredded and frozen in a single layer on a sheet pan, then transferred to an airtight container or freezer bag for long-term storage. Use within 1 year. This is ideal for roots, like horseradish, being used in preparations such as vinegar-based tinctures and oxymels such as fire cider, as well as mucilaginous roots such as marshmallow for cold infusions.

TINCTURING HERBS FOR MEDICINE

While tincturing also qualifies as medicine making, it is important to understand that the act of immersing an herb in alcohol (or chosen menstruum such as glycerin or vinegar) is itself an act of preservation. See page 24 for tincture instructions.

SIMPLE HERBAL REMEDY FORMULAS

My intent with this book was always to set an herbalist and gardener on the path to trusting their intuition and to give one confidence in the preparation of herbal remedies. As such, I have included very few precise remedies. Instead, I invite the reader to use these basic formulas to produce remedies according to the specific needs of the individual based on knowledge earned.

Tea

Teas are the perfect low-dose remedy to offer herbal support for mild complaints, such as the common cold or an upset stomach, and are generally well tolerated even when consumed daily or often throughout a day. This preparation is ideal for delicate leaf- and flower-type plant matter.

1 tablespoon (1–2 g) dried herbs or
2–3 tablespoons (5–10 g) fresh chopped herbs
8–10 ounces (235–295 ml) water, just off the boil

Infuse the herbs in the hot water for 5 to 7 minutes. Strain and serve.

Teas can be consumed as often as two to three times daily.

Hot Infusion

Compared to teas, infusions steep for longer and thus offer a greater extraction of medicinal constituents, as well as flavor and aromatics. Because they deliver stronger herbal medicine, they are ideal for more chronic or irritating complaints, such as menstrual cramping, poor digestion and infection. This type of preparation is ideal for leaf, flower and small root and bark plant matter.

¼–½ cup (5–10 g) dried herbs or ½–1 cup (15–30 g) fresh herbs

16 ounces (475 ml) water, just off the boil

Infuse the herbs in the water for 20 to 30 minutes. Strain and serve. Refrigerate any unused infusion for up to 48 hours.

Consume one to two times daily.

Single-Dose Cold Infusion

This is the perfect remedy utilizing demulcent herbs like marshmallow and licorice for sore throats, dry coughs and those prone to acidic reflux and heartburn. Meant to be taken like a "shot," these single-dose infusions deliver fast relief.

1 heaping teaspoon (1 g) dried herbs or 1 tablespoon (3 g) fresh herbs

2 ounces (60 ml) water

Place the herbs and water into a small glass. Infuse for a minimum of 2 hours. Strain the liquid, discarding the herbs, and take the cold infusion quickly in either a shot or a few sips. This remedy is best prepared fresh due to the mucilage content and infusion time needed.

Single-dose cold infusions can be taken two to three times daily.

Cold Infusion

A cold infusion is ideal when one wants to maximize the delicate flavor and aromatics of herbs, such as rose and honeysuckle, or to minimize tannic and bitter characteristics of herbs like camellia and motherwort.

¼–½ cup (5–10 g) dried herbs or ½–1 cup (15–30 g) fresh herbs

16 ounces (475 ml) water

Infuse the herbs in the water for 12 to 24 hours in a cool spot or the refrigerator. Strain and serve. Refrigerate unused infusion for up to 48 hours.

Cold infusions can be consumed two to three times daily.

Decoction

Decoctions are usually reserved for hardy roots and barks, as well as dried mushrooms. The simmering action provides for thorough extraction of this denser plant material, thus creating a very nutritive, powerful remedy. Decoctions are perfect for addressing deep-seated issues like adrenal fatigue and persistent digestive dysfunction.

2 cups fresh or 1 cup dried (50–150 g depending on the density of the herbal material) roots or bark

32 ounces (945 ml) water

Place the herbs and water in a small saucepan over medium heat and simmer for 20 to 30 minutes or until the volume of water is reduced by half. Remove from the heat, strain and serve. Refrigerate unused decoction for up to 48 hours.

Decoctions should be consumed once daily.

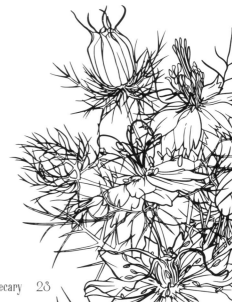

Tincture

Tincturing is a method that leads to great extraction of a variety of medicinal constituents using solvent action. Tincture remedies are one of the more potent medicinal offerings of the home apothecary. With a long shelf life, tinctures are a great remedy to have on hand and they travel well compared to bulk herbs and infusions.

When creating a tincture, one must first choose the appropriate menstruum (the solvent used to extract the medicinal constituents of the herbs used).

Low-Proof Alcohol: *Use vodka or preferred spirits with a proof of 80 (alcohol content of about 40%), for most fresh or dried leaf and flower material.*

Mid-Proof Alcohol: *Vodka with a proof of 100 is appropriate for most leaf, flower and small berry plant material, especially when using fresh herbs (the higher alcohol content prolongs the shelf life).*

High–Mid Alcohol: *Combine one part 100-proof vodka with one part 190-proof distilled spirits to facilitate a strong extraction of barks, thick roots and fleshy berries/fruits, like hawthorn and rose hips.*

High-Proof Alcohol: *Any 190-proof spirit can be used for tough bark, roots and resinous plant materials such as cottonwood buds.*

Vinegar: *Vinegar should be used when desiring a greater extraction of the mineral constituents of certain herbs like nettle. A vinegar-based tincture can be combined with honey to taste to create an oxymel if desired.*

Vegetable Glycerin: *Relatively poor in solvent action, use glycerin when alcohol is being avoided or when the intended remedy is for children (glycerin is sweet). This is best for leaf and floral plant matter. If tincturing more robust plant material, use a blender to break up the herb and maximize the glycerin extraction.*

---

4 ounces (115 g) dried herbs or 6 ounces (170 g) fresh herbs

16 ounces (475 ml) chosen menstruum

Place herbs and menstruum in a jar with a tight-fitting lid. Infuse for 6 to 8 weeks in a cool dark place, shaking daily. Strain using a fine-meshed sieve lined with a layer of muslin, or two layers of cheesecloth. Pour into amber glass bottles outfitted with a dropper. Keep in a cool, dry place for up to 2 years.

Tincture dosing depends on the herb used.

Typical dosages range from 1 to 2 dropperfuls (1 to 2 ml) up to three times daily.

Store tinctures in a cool place out of direct light.

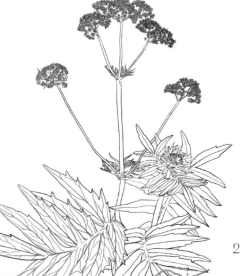

Syrup

A spoonful of sugar helps the medicine go down! This preparation is great for bitter herbs and those being given to children. Simple syrups must be refrigerated, but a heavy syrup is considered shelf stable for up to one year. I generally recommend using organic granulated sugar for syrup preparations as it results in a cleaner flavor and less potential for fermentation. However, feel free to use honey if so desired!

SIMPLE SYRUP

8 ounces (235 ml) water

¼–½ cup (5–10 g) dried herbs or ½ cup (15 g) fresh herbs

8 ounces (227 g) granulated sugar or honey

HEAVY SYRUP

8 ounces (235 ml) water

¼–½ cup (5–10 g) dried herbs or ½ cup (15 g) fresh herbs

16 ounces (455 g) granulated sugar or honey

Combine the water and the herbs in a small saucepan and bring to a gentle boil over medium high heat. Add sugar or honey, stirring until all the sugar is dissolved and then return it to a gentle boil for 1 minute. Remove it from the heat. Once it is cool, strain and pour the syrup into bottles for storage.

Children can benefit from 1 teaspoon (5 ml) of syrup two to three times daily. Adults can typically tolerate 1 tablespoon (15 ml) of syrup three times daily.

Oxymel

Oxymels are an excellent way to deliver pungent and mineral-rich herbal healing, perhaps the most famous of which is fire cider (an oxymel composed of pungent herbs like horseradish, garlic and cayenne, although the preparation varies from maker to maker), but is also particularly useful for maximizing the mineral properties for herbs such as stinging nettle. Oxymels can be taken medicinally, but are also a great base for vinaigrettes or splashed into rich meals like soups and stews for a dose of medicinal acidity.

4 ounces (115 g) dried herbs or 6 ounces (170 g) fresh herbs

16 ounces (475 ml) raw apple cider vinegar

½ cup (118 ml) honey, or to taste

Place the herbs and vinegar in a jar with a tight-fitting lid. Infuse for 6 to 8 weeks in a cool, dark place, shaking daily. Strain using a fine-meshed sieve lined with a layer of muslin, or two layers of cheesecloth. Combine with honey until it is thoroughly incorporated. Pour the oxymel into amber glass bottles outfitted with a dropper. Keep oxymels in a cool, dry place for up to 1 year.

Offer children 1 teaspoon (5 ml) of oxymel two to three times daily. Adults can typically tolerate 1 tablespoon (15 ml) of oxymel three times daily.

Infused Honey

A simple preparation that delights by the dose is an herbally-infused honey. This remedy can be taken by the spoonful for medicinal purposes or even used to top toast or baked goods! It is very important to the shelf stability to use DRIED herbs for this formula.

½ cup (10 g) dried herbs

1 cup (240 ml) honey

Combine the honey and herbs in a jar with a tight-fitting lid. Stir daily or as often as possible and allow this mixture to infuse for 4 to 6 weeks in a relatively warm spot such as a sunny window or near a stove. After the honey has been infused, strain the mixture through a fine-mesh sieve and bottle the honey. Honey can typically be stored indefinitely. If crystallization occurs, place the infused honey container in a bowl of hot water until the honey liquefies.

Children can have 1 teaspoon (5 ml) of infused honey two to three times daily. Adults can enjoy 1 tablespoon (15 ml) of infused honey three times daily.

Honey Fermentation

Fermented honeys are a fun and interesting way to deliver the benefits of herbs and the gut biome benefits of fermentation! This preparation utilizes FRESH herbs that will offer a small amount of liquid that will ignite fermentation. This is a great preparation for fresh rosehips and elderberries but is also wonderful for garlic.

½ cup (10 g) fresh herbs

1 cup (240ml) honey

Place herbs and honey in a jar with at least 1 to 2 inches (2.5 to 5 cm) of headspace. Place a lid on the jar but do not tighten—fermentation will cause a buildup of carbon dioxide pressure that needs to "off gas." Place the jar in a relatively warm spot and stir this mixture daily. As the herbs release moisture, the honey will become runnier and some bubbling can be observed within 1 to 2 weeks. Ferment the herbs and honey for 3 to 4 weeks and strain if desired, but the ferment can be moved to a cool spot for storage with the herbs still in it.

Allow children 1 teaspoon (5 ml) of fermented honey two to three times daily. Adults can indulge in 1 tablespoon (15 ml) of fermented honey three times daily. Freely consume the herbs used for the ferment.

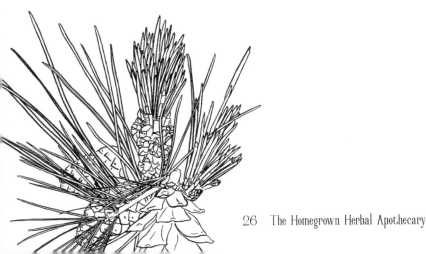

Honey Electuary

Electuaries sound so mysterious but they are little more than a paste crafted from honey and dried, powdered herbs! This enjoyable preparation can be used by the spoonful to create an "instant" sweet herbal tea but can be smeared on bread and baked goods as well! To powder your herbs, use a coffee grinder or a mortar and pestle until the herb is finely granulated.

½ cup (50–60 g) dried powdered herbs

½ cup (240 ml) honey (more or less depending on the desired consistency)

Mix powdered herbs and honey to the desired consistency. Place this in a jar with a tight fitting lid and use within 1 year.

Use your electuary by using a spoonful in hot water for "instant" herbal tea or consume a spoonful as desired!

Oil Infusion

Oil infusions are one of the simplest preparations for skin and body treatments. They are particularly well suited to being used alone as a massage oil or moisturizing body oil. Alternatively, use your medicinal herb-infused oil as a base for a number of other body products, such as salves, lotions and creams.

1 cup (20 g) dried herbs

32 ounces (945 ml) shelf stable oil such as olive oil, coconut oil or jojoba oil

Combine the herbs and oil in a jar with a tight-fitting lid and place it in a warm spot out of direct light to infuse for 6 to 8 weeks. Alternatively, to create a faster oil infusion, this jar can be placed in a slow cooker water bath with the water at least two-thirds up the side of the jar. Keep the water at a stable temperature of 140 to 160°F (60 to 70°C) on low for 2 to 3 days.

After the infusion is complete, strain using a fine-mesh sieve lined with muslin or two layers of cheesecloth. Pour infused oil in an amber glass jar and use it within 1 year.

Salve

Salves are so easy to make and are very useful for addressing a wide variety of wounds such as minor cuts, scrapes and punctures, as well as bruises, sprains and painful joints.

8 ounces (235 ml) herb-infused oil

2–4 tablespoons (18–36 g) beeswax pastilles (depending on how soft or firm the desired salve should be)

In a double boiler, add the infused oil and beeswax. Warm until the wax is completely melted. Remove the oil/beeswax mixture from the heat and pour it into individual 2-ounce (30-ml) containers (approximately four containers) or other similarly-sized jars. Allow it to cool completely before putting a lid on the container. Use within 1 year.

Lotion

Lotions are a great way to revitalize ashy and dehydrated skin. This preparation will result in a light, pumpable lotion perfect for applying to skin. Note: Due to the aqueous quotient of a lotion, this preparation should be used within 2 weeks, stored in the refrigerator or preserved with commercially available preservatives. There are a variety of preservatives on the market, but I have not included them in this recipe as each will have its own suggested use. If not using a preservative, pay close attention for signs of spoilage such as mold or mildew growth, "off" smells or changes in texture.

22 ounces (650 ml) water-based herbal infusion (or some part of this can be aloe vera gel)

8 ounces (235 ml) herb-infused oil

1 ounce (28 g) emulsifying wax pastilles (see Tip)

In a double boiler, heat the infused oil and emulsifying wax until combined. Meanwhile, warm your water-based ingredients to the same approximate temperature as the oil/wax mixture to help the emulsification process.

Remove the oil mixture from the heat and pour it into a medium-sized bowl. Using an immersion blender, handheld mixer or whisk, slowly pour the water-based liquid into the oil, while whisking continuously, until it is emulsified and evenly combined. Pour the mixture into amber glass bottles outfitted with a pump.

— **Tip:** Emulsifying wax has unique properties that help to suspend oil and water. Avoid use of beeswax or other waxes for lotions and creams as they do not have the same binding properties and may result in your emulsification "breaking" or separating.

Cream

For a sumptuous moisture experience, craft an oil-rich cream for dry, crepey skin. Note: Due to the aqueous quotient of a cream, this preparation should be used within 2 weeks, stored in the refrigerator or preserved with a commercially available preservative. There are a variety of preservatives on the market, but I have not included them in this recipe as each will have its own suggested use. If not using a preservative, pay close attention for signs of spoilage such as mold or mildew growth, "off" smells or changes in texture. Always use clean, dry fingers or clean implements such as a cosmetic "spatula" or swab to remove cream from the jar.

2 tablespoons (30 ml) herb-infused oil

2 tablespoons (30 ml) plant-based "butter," such as cocoa, shea, kokum or mango

2 tablespoons (18 g) emulsifying wax pastilles

2 tablespoons (30 ml) specialty oil, such as rose hip, sea buckthorn or evening primrose (or substitute with more herb-infused oil)

6–10 tablespoons (90–150 ml) hydrosol, water-based herbal infusion, aloe, distilled water or a mixture thereof

In a double boiler, heat the herb-infused oil, plant butter and wax pastilles until they are melted and evenly combined. Meanwhile, warm your water-based ingredients to the same approximate temperature of the oil/wax mixture to help the emulsification process.

Pour the oil/wax mixture into a medium-sized bowl. Using an immersion blender, handheld mixer or whisk, slowly pour the water-based ingredient into the oils, while whisking continuously, until evenly combined and your desired consistency is achieved. Pour or pipe into a jar or other container of your choice.

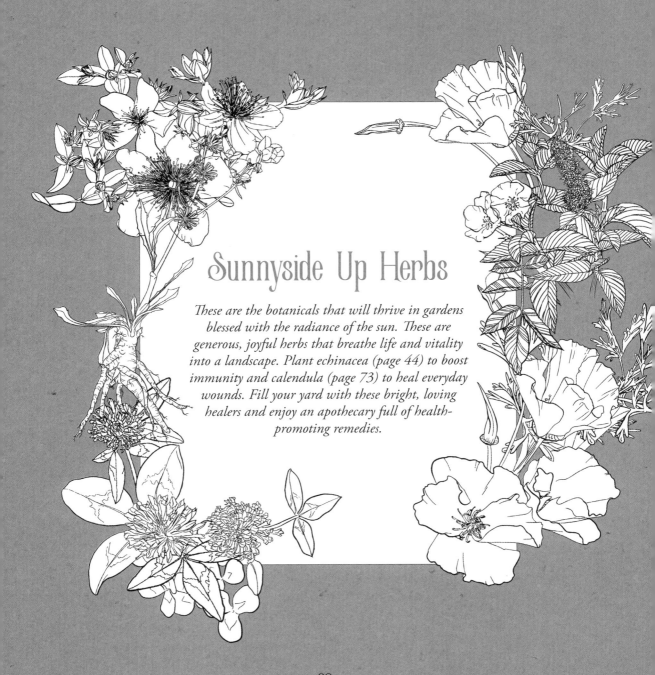

Sunnyside Up Herbs

These are the botanicals that will thrive in gardens blessed with the radiance of the sun. These are generous, joyful herbs that breathe life and vitality into a landscape. Plant echinacea (page 44) to boost immunity and calendula (page 73) to heal everyday wounds. Fill your yard with these bright, loving healers and enjoy an apothecary full of health-promoting remedies.

Borage

Borago officinalis

Herbal Energetics: Cool/moist
Signatures: Courageous, heartening

Borage is a remarkably cooling herb offering a variety of benefits, especially when there are concerns of excessive heat such as fever, inflammation and localized skin irritation. This herb seems to have an affinity for the metaphorical heart and has been used to ease depression and general melancholy while increasing a sense of courage and clarity, perhaps owing these benefits to its positive action on the adrenal system. Additionally, borage is thought to increase lactation, and the oil made from its seeds helps to soften the cervix in preparation for labor. The cooling, demulcent nature of borage also makes it an excellent remedy for sore throat and cough.

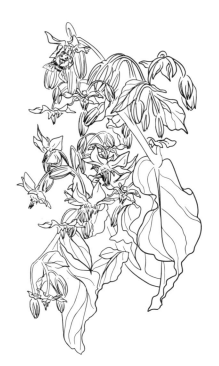

PLANT SNAPSHOT

Annual
Zone: 3–10
Growth Habit: Upright, bushy

GROWING THIS HEALING BOTANICAL

Light Requirements: Full sun

Garden Placement: Borage grows 1 to 3 feet (0.3 to 0.9 m) wide, so make sure you give it plenty of space to grow and reseed.

Soil Preference: Borage adapts to a variety of soil conditions and water supplies, but thrives in moderately fertile, slightly moist, loamy soils.

When to Plant: Sow seeds indoors, 3 to 4 weeks before the last frost under an ascending moon. Plant seedings when danger of frost has passed, under a waning moon.

Best Growing Tips: As an ambitious reseeder, borage is an excellent choice to fill in large blank spots in the garden.

Garden Companions: Borage is a powerful attractor of pollinators, and its cucumber-like scent is thought to deter tomato hornworms, making this an excellent herb to plant in a vegetable patch.

HARVESTING THIS HERBAL ALLY

Parts Used: Leaves, flowers

When to Harvest for Medicinal Potency: Harvest under an ascending moon while the blue star-shaped flowers are blooming.

HERBAL REMEDY TIP

Borage makes an excellent iced tea when combined with spearmint (refer to page 23 for a cold infusion). The cooling properties are perfect for relaxing and unwinding after a day in the sun!

Catmint

Nepeta cataria

Herbal Energetics: Cool/dry
Signatures: Alluring, inviting

Well known for its feline allure, catmint is of great use in the herbal apothecary for its wide-ranging benefits. This profoundly cooling herb reduces body temperature and encourages perspiration, making it a premier remedy for sun exposure, exertion, hot flashes and fever. Catmint acts on the digestive system to relieve complaints of cramping, bloating and flatulence and can even be used to soothe colicky infants. This herb is also a great tool for calming overstimulated and hyperactive children and has gentle sedative action for all.

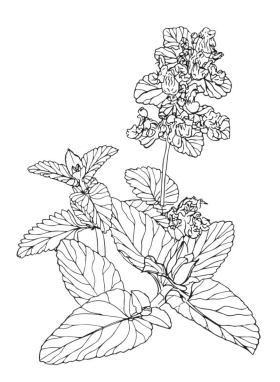

PLANT SNAPSHOT

Perennial
Zone: 3–8
Growth Habit: Bushy, full

GROWING THIS HEALING BOTANICAL

Light Requirements: Full sun

Garden Placement: Catmint will quickly fill in bare spots in the garden, making it a great choice for camouflaging unattractive home foundations and in the middle of beds and borders to take up visual space.

Soil Preference: Catmint prefers dry, moderately fertile, loamy or slightly sandy soil with access to irrigation.

When to Plant: Sow catmint seeds 6 to 8 weeks before the last frost (leaving mostly uncovered because the seeds need light to germinate), during a waxing moon.

Best Growing Tips: Like many mint family herbs, catmint is a "cut and come again" plant, so it responds well to being harvested during its first flush of blooms and will likely produce successive harvests throughout the season.

Garden Companions: Plant catmint with lavender, rosemary, salvias and lamb's ear. Catmint may also help to deter common rose pests.

HARVESTING THIS HERBAL ALLY

Parts Used: Leaves, flowers

When to Harvest for Medicinal Potency: Gather growing tips frequently throughout the growing season during a waxing moon.

HERBAL REMEDY TIP

Catmint iced tea is a perfect summer treat. Create a strong infusion (page 22), but instead of using water right off the boil, let it cool slightly until it is very warm before infusing, to preserve the herb's flavor. To make your iced tea, simply dilute the infusion with cold water to taste. This is a perfect sipper after a hot day to ease you into a good night's sleep.

Eyebright

Euphrasia officinalis

Herbal Energetics: Cool/dry
Signatures: Clear, glowing

As the name suggests, this petite botanical is a perfect remedy for a variety of eye complaints. The cooling, toning nature of eyebright soothes the inflamed tissues around the eye. The herb aids in complaints of itchy, watery eyes, conjunctivitis, styes and blepharitis. Not limited to the treatment of eyes, as a natural antihistamine, eyebright is a remedy for seasonal allergy complaints, such as a running nose, itchy skin and cough.

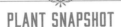

PLANT SNAPSHOT

Annual
Zone: 1–9
Growth Habit: Low-growing

GROWING THIS HEALING BOTANICAL

Light Requirements: Full sun

Garden Placement: Plant in masses toward the front of a border.

Soil Preference: Eyebright is adaptive to a variety of soil fertility and prefers well-drained soil.

When to Plant: This botanical requires cold stratification in order to germinate, so sow seeds in mid-fall under an ascending moon.

Best Growing Tips: A native to grassy meadows, this is a great herb to grow in areas where grass is patchy and sparse.

Garden Companions: Plant among native grasses and clovers for a naturalized meadow.

HARVESTING THIS HERBAL ALLY

Parts Used: Leaves, flowers

When to Harvest for Medicinal Potency: Gather leaves and flowers throughout the bloom cycle under a waxing moon.

HERBAL REMEDY TIP

For red, itchy eyes, prepare an infusion (page 22) with eyebright and allow it to cool. Soak cotton disks in the cooled infusion and place them on the eyes.

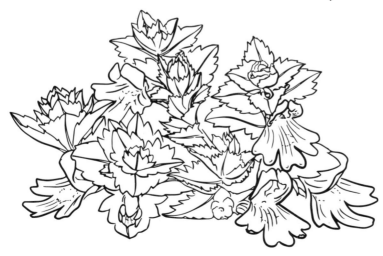

Feverfew

Tanacetum parthenium

Herbal Energetics: Cool/dry
Signatures: Pervasive, insistent, joyful

As its common name implies, this is an herb with a heralded reputation for reducing fever. Feverfew also has profound anti-inflammatory and pain-relieving properties, making it a proper, natural remedy for rheumatoid arthritis sufferers. It is also a popular botanical for addressing migraines. Consistent, regular use of feverfew may help to decrease migraine occurrence and reduce the severity of acute symptoms. Applied topically, feverfew is a natural insect repellent.

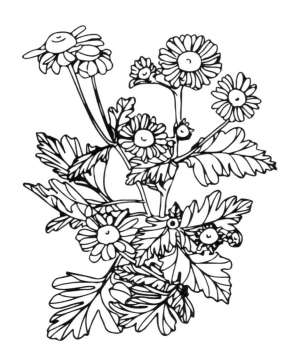

PLANT SNAPSHOT

Perennial
Zone: 5–10
Growth Habit: Full, mounding

GROWING THIS HEALING BOTANICAL

Light Requirements: Full sun to partial shade

Garden Placement: Grow feverfew toward the middle or back of borders and beds as it reaches approximately 2 feet (0.6 m) in height and can be quite full.

Soil Preference: Feverfew prefers soils rich in organic matter but are generally unfussy after well established.

When to Plant: Sow seeds directly outdoors in spring while the soil is still damp, pressing them into the soil surface but not covering them, under a waxing moon cycle.

Best Growing Tips: Feverfew creates beautiful drifts of petite, daisy-like flowers that last all summer long. Plant in mass or undulating lines throughout beds to bring a pop of brightness and accentuate darker flowers and foliage.

Garden Companions: As a natural insect repellent, grow feverfew near prone and susceptible plants such as roses and brassica family vegetables.

HARVESTING THIS HERBAL ALLY

Parts Used: Leaves, flowers

When to Harvest for Medicinal Potency: Harvest leaves and flowers under an ascending moon.

HERBAL REMEDY TIP

Feverfew teaches migraine sufferers the importance of consistent self-care. When taken daily as a tincture (page 24), this herb can help prevent the severity, duration and frequency of challenging migraine symptoms.

Mullein

Verbascum thapsus

Herbal Energetics: Cool/dry
Signatures: Tender, gentle, uplifting

The soft fuzzy leaves, towering stance and tiny ear-like flowers of mullein are a lesson in the doctrine of signatures. Mullein leaves are a remedy for the lungs and throat and is a favored treatment for irritation caused by inhalation of particulate matter, hardened phlegm and an unproductive cough. The stem and roots are thought to support the spine and connective tissues of the body, increasing flexibility and range of motion, especially after injury. The petite flowers have been used for centuries to address earaches and tender lymphatic tissue near the neck.

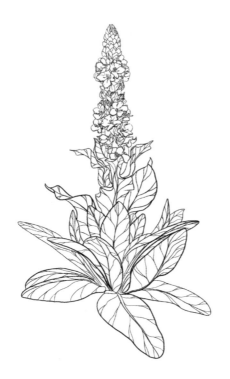

PLANT SNAPSHOT

Biennial
Zone: 3–9
Growth Habit: Towering, upright

GROWING THIS HEALING BOTANICAL

Light Requirements: Full sun

Garden Placement: Mullein can reach heights of 4 to 6 feet (1.2 to 1.8 m), so this botanical is best placed near the back of a border.

Soil Preference: Mullein prefers well-drained soils with access to water but will not tolerate boggy conditions. Mullein thrives in relatively poor and neglected soils.

When to Plant: Mullein seeds should be sown mid-fall to allow for natural cold stratification.

Best Growing Tips: Adaptive mullein grows well in neglected spaces, making it a great selection for carefree spots. Although considered a "weed" by some standards, its silvery foliage and impressive height make it at home in a cottage-inspired garden.

Garden Companions: Plant mullein with echinacea where they can enjoy similar conditions and attract pollinators to a nearby garden patch.

HARVESTING THIS HERBAL ALLY

Parts Used: Leaves, stem, roots, flowers

When to Harvest for Medicinal Potency: Dig first-year roots in early fall or the following spring during a descending moon. The leaves and stalk can be harvested throughout the summer months, while flowers should be gathered in bloom during a waxing moon.

HERBAL REMEDY TIP

Make an oil infusion (page 27) with mullein and keep a bottle of the infused oil in your medicine cabinet for sudden earaches. This is an absolute must-have for addressing acute ear pain when little ones are plagued—always inconveniently late at night!

Sage

Salvia officinalis

Herbal Energetics: Cool/dry
Signatures: Robust, undaunted

Most often thought of as a culinary herb, sage is a cooling, calming powerhouse in the apothecary. Sage is a first choice when there are complaints of hot flashes, overheating from exertion or exposure, fever or just those folks that run HOT. This is the herb to turn to when one is prone to flushing and redness in the skin. Sage is also thought to promote good cognition and improve memory and clarity. This herb is also used to aid in the digestion of fatty foods—perhaps why it is often used to flavor rich holiday fare. One can also find relief from hoarseness and sore throat by gargling a strong infusion of this botanical.

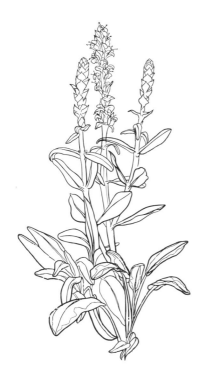

PLANT SNAPSHOT

Perennial
Zone: 5–9
Growth Habit: Mounding, woody

GROWING THIS HEALING BOTANICAL

Light Requirements: Full sun

Garden Placement: This fairly low-growing botanical is at home at the front of borders or in pots. Different varieties boast yellow and purple tones, adding visual interest to potted arrangements.

Soil Preference: Sage prefers light sandy soils that are modest in fertility.

When to Plant: Sow sage seeds indoors 6 to 8 weeks before last frost during a waxing moon cycle. Transplant outdoors when danger of frost has passed, under a descending moon.

Best Growing Tips: Sage loves a little heat and tolerates drier, slightly sandy soils, making it a great addition to a xeriscaped garden.

Garden Companions: Plant sage with rosemary and thyme or with cruciferous family veggies or carrots.

HARVESTING THIS HERBAL ALLY

Parts Used: Leaves

When to Harvest for Medicinal Potency: Gather leaves throughout the growing season under an ascending moon.

HERBAL REMEDY TIP

While an enjoyable herb in a variety of culinary applications, sage is also a fast-acting herb for concerns of heat and digestion when used in tincture form (page 24).

Garlic

Allium sativum

Herbal Energetics: Warm/moist
Signatures: Pungent, bold, striking

Possibly one of the most powerful herbs of the kitchen and apothecary alike, garlic is in a class of its own due to ease of use, accessibility and affordability. One of the few classic herbal remedies that has been extensively researched, garlic has great benefits for the cardiovascular system, including its ability to prevent oxidative damage to cells, lower blood pressure and reduce cholesterol levels. Additionally, this pungent herb is profoundly antimicrobial, supporting the immune system in the fight against bacterial, viral and fungal threats.

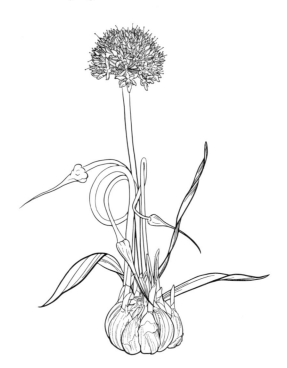

PLANT SNAPSHOT

Perennial, but grown as an annual bulb
Zone: 3–8
Growth Habit: Tall, strap-like

GROWING THIS HEALING BOTANICAL

Light Requirements: Full sun

Garden Placement: Since garlic is primarily harvested as a bulb, grow garlic in an area where it is easily accessed from digging.

Soil Preference: Moderately rich, well-drained loamy soils that retain some moisture without becoming boggy are best for growing garlic.

When to Plant: Plant individual garlic cloves in early fall under a descending moon.

Best Growing Tips: Decide between softneck or hardneck varieties, or grow beds of both. Hardnecks produce a flavorful, flowering scape and larger cloves, while softneck varieties are lauded for their ease of storage and ability to braid.

Garden Companions: Garlic is a great deterrent of garden pests and is a welcome addition to a vegetable garden.

HARVESTING THIS HERBAL ALLY

Parts Used: Bulb, scape from hardnecks (edible)

When to Harvest for Medicinal Potency: Harvest bulbs in early summer near the solstice under a descending moon.

HERBAL REMEDY TIP

Garlic cannot be overlooked for its medicinal benefits in everyday foods. However, my favorite potent remedy is to create a honey fermentation (page 26) using fresh garlic cloves in honey. Eat a clove and/or take a spoonful of the infused honey at the first sign of impending illness.

Angelica

Angelica archangelica

Herbal Energetics: Warm/dry
Signatures: Spicy, inviting

Angelica is an intensely aromatic and incredibly stimulating herb perfect for remedying cold, stagnant conditions. This botanical is ideal for those feeling clammy and sluggish and is particularly good for breaking a low-grade fever that is coupled with sore, achy joints. Angelica can also loosen deep lung congestion and lift a sense of heaviness in the chest. It can be used to bring on a delayed menstruation and address chronic amenorrhea, while also easing cramping before a period. It is a wonderful carminative herb that greatly reduces bloating, indigestion and flatulence.

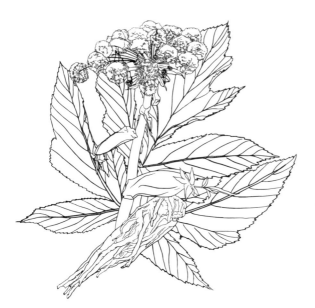

PLANT SNAPSHOT

Short-lived perennial
Zone: 4–9
Growth Habit: Upright

GROWING THIS HEALING BOTANICAL

Light Requirements: Full sun to partial shade

Garden Placement: The blooming stems of angelica can grow up to 3 feet (0.9 m) tall and is best placed toward the middle or back of a bed or border.

Soil Preference: The long taproot of angelica requires loose, well-drained soil of average fertility to thrive. Give angelica ample moisture while establishing; more mature plants appreciate drier conditions.

When to Plant: Sow angelica seeds directly into prepared soil in the fall to allow for cold stratification and to minimize handling and damage of the taproot while transplanting.

Best Growing Tips: Angelica is fairly short-lived and biennial in nature with some conditions. As such, it is best to sow fresh seeds each year to keep a perpetual supply on hand!

Garden Companions: Underplant angelica with sweet woodruff to keep the soil cool.

HARVESTING THIS HERBAL ALLY

Parts Used: Root (Note: Leaves, stems and seeds are edible but not often used medicinally.)

When to Harvest for Medicinal Potency: Dig up roots in early fall during a descending moon.

HERBAL REMEDY TIP

A tea (page 22) of angelica root is excellent for boggy lung conditions and indigestion, while a tincture (page 24) can act swiftly on menstrual complaints.

Dill

Anethum graveolens

Herbal Energetics: Warm/dry
Signatures: Uplifting

Not just the culinary herb used to flavor pickles, dill is an outstanding apothecary herb, especially for stomach complaints. Dill curbs nausea and stimulates the appetite while also reducing cramping, bloating and gas. It has the incredible ability to stop fits of hiccups almost immediately and can be used for colicky infants. Dill can also be used to alleviate menstrual cramping and relieve tenderness in the bladder. It is also a relaxing herb that uplifts spirits.

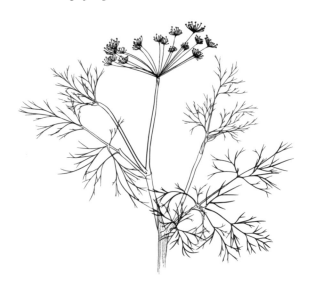

PLANT SNAPSHOT
Annual
Zone: 3–11
Growth Habit: Upright

GROWING THIS HEALING BOTANICAL

Light Requirements: Full sun

Garden Placement: Plant dill near the back of borders and beds and near vegetable patches to attract pollinators.

Soil Preference: Dill likes moderately fertile loam and well-drained soils.

When to Plant: Sow dill seeds directly into prepared soil in mid-fall or early spring when the weather is cool during an ascending moon.

Best Growing Tips: Avoid overhead watering as dill can be prone to rot and is intolerant of humidity.

Garden Companions: Dill makes a great companion for cucumbers, corn and asparagus.

HARVESTING THIS HERBAL ALLY

Parts Used: Leaves, seeds

When to Harvest for Medicinal Potency: Gather leaves throughout the growing season during an ascending moon. Dill seeds can be collected as they start to feel dry to the touch.

HERBAL REMEDY TIP

A simple pinch of dill seeds eaten plain is the perfect remedy to grab in a bind for instances of hiccups and indigestion.

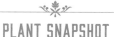

Fennel

Foeniculum vulgare

Herbal Energetics: Warm/moist
Signatures: Strong yet delicate

This anise-flavored, licorice-y herb is a gentle antispasmodic known for its digestive benefits. Fennel is a favored remedy for that too-full, eyes bigger than my plate type feeling. Additionally, it is a wonderful herb for stomach cramping, gas and nausea. Fennel is also a great herb to add as an adjunct herb for menstrual complaints and can increase milk flow in nursing mothers.

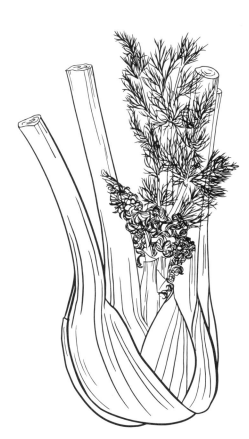

PLANT SNAPSHOT

Biennial
Zone: 4–9
Growth Habit: Upright

GROWING THIS HEALING BOTANICAL

Light Requirements: Full sun

Garden Placement: Fennel is most at home near the back of a border where it has a place to reseed and flourish.

Soil Preference: This botanical prefers fertile, well-drained, loamy soils

When to Plant: Sow fennel seeds indoors 4 to 6 weeks before the last frost or outdoors after the danger of frost has past under a new or waxing moon.

Best Growing Tips: Fennel has a reputation for being slightly allelopathic, meaning it can inhibit the growth of nearby plants. Give this herb a spot of its own with room to grow.

Garden Companions: Due to its allelopathic properties, fennel does not play well with others but is a powerful attractor of pollinators. As such, it is a great option for containers. However, I have found that diverse herbs with low water and fertility requirements such as rosemary and lavender can tolerate proximity to this botanical.

HARVESTING THIS HERBAL ALLY

Parts Used: Bulb, stems, leaves, flowers, seeds

When to Harvest for Medicinal Potency: Harvest leaves and flowers under an ascending moon throughout the growing season. Bulbs taste best when the weather cools and can be harvested under a waxing moon. Gather seeds when they are dry to the touch.

HERBAL REMEDY TIP

I enjoy fennel greatly in meals and teas, but sometimes a simple remedy is all that you need. Keep a small dish of dried fennel seeds on the table to chew after a sizable feast to aid digestion!

Horehound

Marrubium vulgare

Herbal Energetics: Cool/dry
Signatures: Adaptive, persistent

This intensely bitter herb is widely used for concerns of the respiratory and digestive systems. Horehound promotes the flow of mucosal secretion, so as such it is used for complaints of thick, unproductive cough, deep congestion and intense sinus pressure. The botanical also aids the digestive system by encouraging the salivary response, soothing esophageal and stomach tissues irritated by acid reflux and assisting in the digestion of fat.

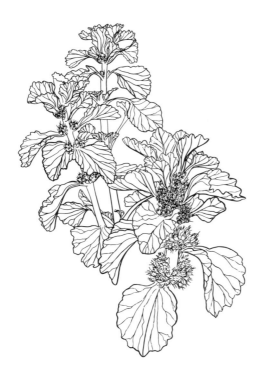

PLANT SNAPSHOT

Perennial
Zone: 3–9
Growth Habit: Branching, bushy

GROWING THIS HEALING BOTANICAL

Light Requirements: Full sun

Garden Placement: Reaching a height of about 18 to 24 inches (46 to 61 cm) tall, this herb should be planted in the middle of a bed or border, or along a fence line with room to spread.

Soil Preference: Horehound prefers somewhat dry, well-drained soils of poor to moderate fertility.

When to Plant: Sow seeds indoors, approximately 4 to 6 weeks before last frost under a waxing moon cycle.

Best Growing Tips: As a member of the mint family, give horehound plenty of room to "roam" or plant in a pot to keep it contained.

Garden Companions: Horehound stimulates the fruiting of nightshades such as tomatoes and peppers.

HARVESTING THIS HERBAL ALLY

Parts Used: Leaves, flowers

When to Harvest for Medicinal Potency: Gather flowering stems throughout the growing season under an ascending moon.

HERBAL REMEDY TIP

Due to the bitter nature of horehound, this remedy is most palatable when consumed as a syrup (page 25).

Mint

Mentha species (Mentha piperita, spicata)

Herbal Energetics: Cool/dry
Signatures: Adaptive, accommodating, generous

Familiar to virtually everyone, mint is a beloved herb. Medicinally speaking, peppermint and spearmint are some of the most widely used members of the mint family. Many herbalists find peppermint especially soothing for the gastrointestinal tract, and it is a chief remedy for complaints of nausea, motion sickness and indigestion. Spearmint is thought to have a more pronounced action on the respiratory system, helping to open airways and loosen phlegm. Mints tend to encourage perspiration and can be a very gentle remedy for breaking high fevers.

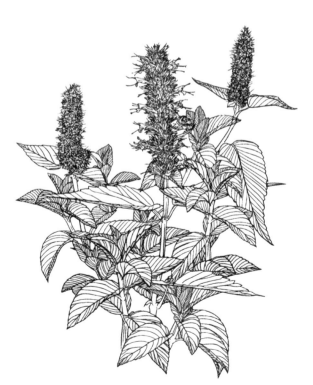

PLANT SNAPSHOT

Perennial
Zone: 3–8
Growth Habit: Vigorous, upright

GROWING THIS HEALING BOTANICAL

Light Requirements: Full sun to light shade

Garden Placement: Members of the mint family will quickly fill in bare areas of the garden and should be grown near where it can be harvested frequently. Plant in containers to control the spread of this botanical.

Soil Preference: Mints tend to prefer moderately rich, well-drained, loamy soils.

When to Plant: Sow seeds indoors, 8 to 10 weeks before last frost during an ascending moon. Transplant outdoors after the danger of frost has passed, under a waning moon.

Best Growing Tips: Mint is so carefree that it is the perfect botanical for spots that you wish to cover ground, control soil erosion and bring color to. Just know that once you plant a bit of mint, you will have it forever!

Garden Companions: Mint family members are excellent choices for planting in the vegetable patch as they attract beneficial pollinators and deter unwanted garden pests!

HARVESTING THIS HERBAL ALLY

Parts Used: Leaves, flowering tips

When to Harvest for Medicinal Potency: Gather leaves and flowering tips throughout the growing season during a waxing moon.

HERBAL REMEDY TIP

A simple mint tea (page 22) sipped any time of day can calm a nervous stomach and uplift the spirits! Another favored remedy for reducing a fever in a small child is to soak socks in a mint infusion (page 22) that has cooled, place the damp socks on the feet, layer with dry ones and let the natural cooling bring down the fevered state!

Peach

Prunus persica

Herbal Energetics: Cool/damp
Signatures: Hydrating, generous

In addition to its generous fruits, the peach tree offers an abundance of medicinal benefits. Another study in the doctrine of signatures, peach is a cooling, moistening herb, of which the myriad benefits few understand. Peach is an ideal remedy for complaints of redness, irritation and dryness when summer allergies persist. Peach tree is a specific herb called for when morning sickness and nausea present in an otherwise hot and dry person. This is an herb to turn to when hot, dry, irritative conditions are persistent!

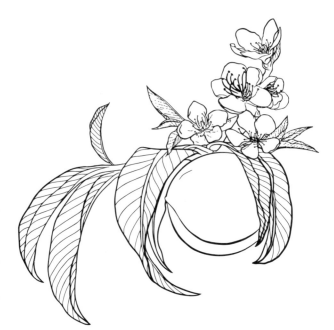

PLANT SNAPSHOT
Tree
Zone: 4–9
Growth Habit: Upright, encompassing

GROWING THIS HEALING BOTANICAL

Light Requirements: Full sun

Garden Placement: Plant near the back of a border or in fruitful hedgerows for maximum effect.

Soil Preference: Plant peach trees in light, rich soils where they are well drained.

When to Plant: Soak peach pits overnight and then place them in damp potting soil for a period of 1 to 3 months, until roots sprout. Transplant seedlings or established trees under a descending moon after the danger of frost has passed.

Best Growing Tips: Young peach trees need ample water during the first couple of years and respond well to pruning to open the canopy.

Garden Companions: Underplanting peach trees with garlic or onions may help deter peach pests.

HARVESTING THIS HERBAL ALLY

Parts Used: Leaves, fruit (edible)

When to Harvest for Medicinal Potency: Harvest leaves throughout the growing season under a waxing moon. Fruit can be picked at the height of ripeness.

HERBAL REMEDY TIP

Fresh peach leaf tincture (page 24) is ideal for cooling down hot, inflamed, acute conditions and morning sickness with frequent vomiting.

Chives

Allium schoenoprasum

Herbal Energetics: Warm/damp
Signatures: Pungent, upright, bold

Far from only a tasty garnish, chives offer a variety of health benefits. Like other members of the allium family, this botanical is full of powerful antioxidants that ward off cell damage and may be particularly good for preventing and addressing gastrointestinal infections. Additionally, chives are full of calcium and vitamin K, making this herb a great choice to support bone health. This herb is a powerful promoter of heart health due to its allicin and potassium content, which helps maintain healthy cholesterol levels and great circulation.

PLANT SNAPSHOT

Perennial
Zone: 3–9
Growth Habit: Upright, vase shaped

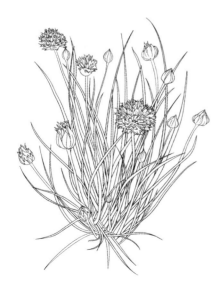

GROWING THIS HEALING BOTANICAL

Light Requirements: Full sun to partial shade

Garden Placement: This long-lived perennial is perfect toward the front of a border and is a great element placed next to lower growing and trailing herbs.

Soil Preference: Chives prefer well-drained, loamy soil with rich fertility.

When to Plant: Sow seeds indoors 6 to 8 weeks before the last frost, or outdoors 4 to 6 weeks before last frost. Unlike many other seeds, chives need complete darkness to germinate, so planting during a waning moon can aid their development. Transplant to the garden when the chives are 4 to 6 inches (10 to 15 cm) tall under a descending moon.

Best Growing Tips: Chives flourish in the garden, providing texture, movement and the loveliest pink-lavender bloom. Plant where they can be easily accessed by the kitchen for frequent harvests of the tips.

Garden Companions: One for the best vegetable and strawberry patch companions, chives deter a variety of pests and attract pollinators.

HARVESTING THIS HERBAL ALLY

Parts Used: Stalks, flowers

When to Harvest for Medicinal Potency: Harvest throughout the growing season for daily meals. Harvest flowers as they open under a waxing moon cycle.

HERBAL REMEDY TIP

Of course, snipping chive tips to flavor foods is an easy way to get the benefits of this herb any time. But for something truly special, infuse white wine or rice vinegar with the blossom (follow the method for a cold infusion on page 23, using vinegar in place of water). Use the infused vinegar to bring an antioxidant rich splash of acidity to dishes, make homemade salad dressings or use as a base for an oxymel (page 25).

Echinacea

Echinacea angustifolia, purpurea, pallida

Herbal Energetics: Warm to cool/dry
Signatures: Determined, tenacious

Perhaps one of the most celebrated immune system supporting herbs, echinacea is an ally for wellness. The initial taste of this botanical is hot and acrid, producing a numbing effect on the mouth and throat, but resolves to a net cooling effect on the body. Echinacea encourages salivation, thus increasing oral and digestive health. Considered an alterative herb, echinacea induces phagocytosis, a lymphatic process of removing microbes, damaged cells and metabolic wastes in the body— and it is this action to which it owes a great deal of its immune system benefits.

PLANT SNAPSHOT

Perennial
Zone: 4–9
Growth Habit: Upright, open

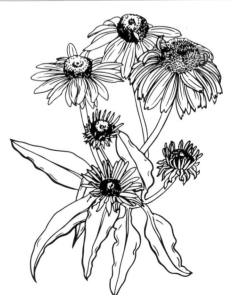

GROWING THIS HEALING BOTANICAL

Light Requirements: Full sun

Garden Placement: Growing 2 to 5 feet (0.6 to 1.5 m) tall, echinacea is best planted toward the middle to back of an ornamental border but is particularly impressive when planted at a large mass to create a blanket of the repeating blooms.

Soil Preference: Well-drained soils of moderate fertility, preferably with a slightly acidic pH.

When to Plant: Echinacea seeds require cold stratification for good germination, so they are best sown directly into the garden in fall so they experience winter freezes. Alternatively, dampen seeds, seal in a container and refrigerate them for 8 to 10 weeks, before starting the seeds under a waning moon. Transplant seedlings outdoors mid-spring under a descending moon.

Best Growing Tips: A native of the prairie states and provinces of North America, echinacea is hardy and drought tolerant, making it an excellent choice for drier garden areas.

Garden Companions: Plant with fellow immune system ally goldenrod, which shares similar growing requirements, for a stunning display of color.

HARVESTING THIS HERBAL ALLY

Parts Used: Roots, leaves, flowers

When to Harvest for Medicinal Potency: Harvest leaves and flowers throughout the growing system from well-established plants (1 to 2 years old), during a waxing moon. Roots should be harvested in late summer under a descending moon.

HERBAL REMEDY TIP

While the roots have been considered the most medicinally valuable, many herbalists subscribe to the notion that the whole plant serves greater healing potential. I like to create a leaf and flower tincture during the summer and a root tincture (page 24) in early fall for maximum efficacy.

Chicory

Cichorium intybus

Herbal Energetics: Cool/dry
Signatures: Wild, pervasive

While often roasted and used as a coffee substitute, chicory is so much more than a caffeine-free cup of "joe." Chicory has an affinity for the liver, stomach and kidneys. It is a gentle diuretic, providing urinary tract relief especially when the bladder never feels fully emptied. Considered a blood purifier, chicory is an excellent detoxifier and may also have benefits for enlarged or fatty liver complaints. Additionally, chicory helps to neutralize stomach acid, making it an excellent choice after meals.

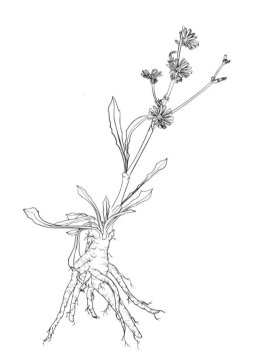

PLANT SNAPSHOT

Biennial
Zone: 3–10
Growth Habit: Feathery, open

GROWING THIS HEALING BOTANICAL

Light Requirements: Full sun

Garden Placement: Growing 2 to 3 feet (0.6 to 0.9 m) tall, chicory is a carefree botanical best suited for wildflower patches.

Soil Preference: Chicory prefers open, well-drained soils with modest fertility.

When to Plant: Sow seeds in early spring directly into the soil with a fine layer of mulch to keep seeds moist under an ascending moon.

Best Growing Tips: I treat this herb as a wild-flower and like to establish it in carefree borders. Its long, slender taproot and adaptive nature will help it reseed and return year after year. As a biennial, it may not flower its first year.

Garden Companions: Chicory grows well with root crops such as beets and radishes and may also help deter garden pests from strawberries and cucumbers.

HARVESTING THIS HERBAL ALLY

Parts Used: Leaves, flowers, roots

When to Harvest for Medicinal Potency: Gather leaves and flowers for edible purposes during a waxing moon phase throughout the blooming season. Harvest taproots in late summer and early fall under a descending moon.

HERBAL REMEDY TIP

I love enjoying a cup of roasted chicory "coffee," prepared as a decoction (page 23). Roast dry roots in a cast iron pan on the stove top over medium-high heat or in the oven at 475°F (220°C), stirring often to achieve even browning. Cool the roasted chicory root and store it until you are ready to prepare the decoction. Its soothing nature makes it a perfect beverage after a large meal and relieves that sense of fullness that can hinder sleep.

Cornsilk

Zea mays

Herbal Energetics: Cool/moist
Signatures: Towering, bountiful

A much-loved member of the vegetable garden, corn is an adored treat for the table. Beyond its value as a food source, the cornsilk is a wonderful remedy for the renal and urinary systems. This botanical is used for concerns such as kidney stones, bladder infections, cystitis and problematic prostates. It is also considered a gentle remedy for bedwetting in small children, as it assists with full bladder elimination. Additionally, cornsilks are thought to have positive benefits on the cardiovascular system.

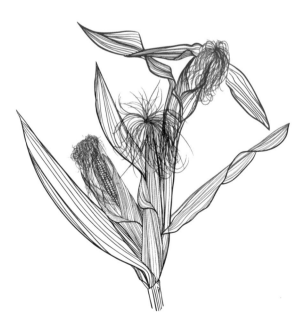

PLANT SNAPSHOT
Annual
Zone: 3–11
Growth Habit: Tall, narrow, upright

GROWING THIS HEALING BOTANICAL

Light Requirements: Full sun

Garden Placement: Plant in a fertile garden spot where it can receive adequate air circulation but be protected from harsh winds.

Soil Preference: Corn likes fertile, well-drained, loamy soils that receive plentiful moisture throughout the growing season.

When to Plant: Plant corn directly in the garden after all danger of frost has passed under an ascending moon.

Best Growing Tips: Corn is considered a heavy feeder and requires a nutrient rich site to flourish.

Garden Companions: Grow corn in the "three sisters" method, with green beans and pumpkins or winter squash as these botanicals create a perfect symbiotic relationship for one another.

HARVESTING THIS HERBAL ALLY

Parts Used: Silks

When to Harvest for Medicinal Potency: Harvest corn under a waxing moon, saving the silks while shucking.

HERBAL REMEDY TIP

I love to use cornsilk as a gentle tea (page 22) with a tiny bit of honey to sweeten. Its wholesome flavor is mild but soothing.

Queen Anne's Lace/ Wild Carrot

Daucus carota

Herbal Energetics: Cool/dry
Signatures: Ethereal

Wild carrot is a strong medicinal ally for the digestive and urinary tracts. Immature seeds are considered greatly carminative—offering relief from gas, bloating and indigestion. As a diuretic, this botanical is helpful for urinary retention, cystitis, bladder infection and may even encourage the expulsion of kidney stones. Additionally, wild carrot is considered a specific herb to address women's reproductive health: toning the uterus, reducing excessive menstrual flow and preventing clotting. It is even suggested for natural family planning. Wild carrot is also used for wound care, particularly that of oozy blisters and sores.

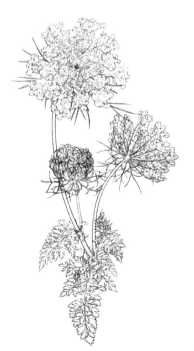

PLANT SNAPSHOT
Biennial
Zone: 4–8
Growth Habit: Open, lacy

GROWING THIS HEALING BOTANICAL

Light Requirements: Full sun

Garden Placement: Wild carrot is most impressive planted in mass and is well suited to unkept roadsides and dry, grassy meadows.

Soil Preference: This botanical prefers well-drained soils and can thrive in poor soil conditions.

When to Plant: In true wildflower form, sow wild carrot seeds in fall and cover them with a thin layer of soil.

Best Growing Tips: Due to the long taproot, if left undisturbed, wild carrot will thrive in areas where other plants suffer. As such, this is an herb to plant in untended areas and be left to flourish on its own.

Garden Companions: This carefree wildflower can benefit lettuces, salad greens and brassica crops by deterring garden pests.

HARVESTING THIS HERBAL ALLY

Parts Used: Flowers, immature (green) seeds

When to Harvest for Medicinal Potency: Gather flowers during an ascending moon throughout the growing season. Harvest seeds when the spent flower forms a "cage," while the seeds are still green during a waxing moon.

HERBAL REMEDY TIP

A pinch of dried green seeds can be chewed to reduce discomfort from eating too much. Sipping wild carrot tea (page 22) during a particularly uncomfortable menstrual cycle can relieve complaints and be an excellent form of simple self-care.

Artichoke

Cynara cardunculus var. scolymus

Herbal Energetics: Cool/moist
Signatures: Cleansing, nutritive, supportive, upright

Like its thistle siblings, the artichoke is an herb that primarily supports wellness by means of detoxification. Artichokes have an affinity for the liver and as such are particularly helpful for hepatic conditions such as heartburn, hangover, hepatitis and bile flow obstruction. As a cleansing herb, this ally also aids to clear the skin, particularly when plagued with hormonal and cystic acne. As the liver also serves a major role in cardiovascular function, artichoke also helps to regulate cholesterol levels. It is also an herb to aid digestion, particularly for those who have trouble tolerating fats and certain proteins.

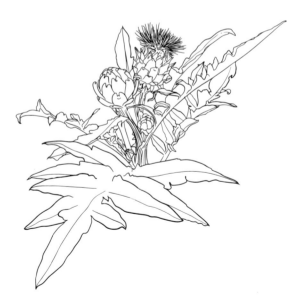

PLANT SNAPSHOT

Perennial
Zone: 7–11
Growth Habit: Upright, vase-shaped, striking

GROWING THIS HEALING BOTANICAL

Light Requirements: Full sun

Garden Placement: Artichokes thrive when given ample room for the roots system to expand to support the substantial plant. Plant near the back of a perennial bed or as impressive "gateway" plants to flank the entry to a garden space.

Soil Preference: Artichokes require fertile soils and benefit from compost additions throughout the growing season. Artichokes prefer well-draining, loamy soils.

When to Plant: Artichoke seeds should be planted indoors 8 to 10 weeks before the last projected frost under a waxing moon. Transplant outdoors when nighttime temperatures are mild under a full or waxing moon.

Best Growing Tips: Artichokes require space. These architectural plants are showiest and happiest when given breathing room.

Garden Companions: Artichokes don't want to complete for nutrients, so plant them near cabbage and other brassica members, peas and even sunflowers to diversify and enhance your garden.

HARVESTING THIS HERBAL ALLY

Parts Used: Leaves, flower, seeds

When to Harvest for Medicinal Potency: Harvest globes throughout the growing season before they start to open for edible purposes. Gather leaves during an ascending moon.

HERBAL REMEDY TIP

A tincture (page 24) of artichoke leaves can be added to a long-term detoxification process, especially when healing from alcoholism and addiction.

Coriander

Coriandrum sativum

Herbal Energetics: Warm (seeds), cool/dry (leaves)

Signatures: Delicate, fine, gentle

Also known as cilantro in its fresh herb form, coriander is a pungent herb known extensively for its detoxification benefits. Although some people are averse to the flavor for culinary purposes, finding it "soapy" tasting, the herbalist will find this herb to be helpful to assist the body in the detoxification of heavy metals. Additionally, it has profound action on the digestive system, in both leaf and seed form, helping to dispel gas, increase appetite and relieve indigestion. Seeds are a great choice for use in both herbal and culinary preparations to clear excessive mucus in the digestive and respiratory systems.

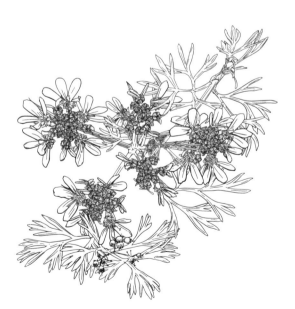

PLANT SNAPSHOT

Free-seeding annual
Zone: 2–10
Growth Habit: Low growing, mounding

GROWING THIS HEALING BOTANICAL

Light Requirements: Full sun with late afternoon shade to delay or prevent its tendency to bolt in hot conditions.

Garden Placement: Plant near the kitchen where the leaves and stems can be trimmed for flavoring meals.

Soil Preference: Coriander likes somewhat moist but well-drained soils of rich fertility.

When to Plant: As taprooted herbs, coriander prefers to be sown directly into containers or gardens. Plant seeds during early spring under an ascending moon and sow seeds successively every 2 to 3 weeks for multiple harvests.

Best Growing Tips: Considered a "shoulder season" botanical, coriander prefers the cooler weather of spring and early fall.

Garden Companions: Plant coriander with other umbellifer family herbs such as dill and fennel, as well as other herbs that prefer moister soil such as basil and parsley.

HARVESTING THIS HERBAL ALLY

Parts Used: Leaves, stems, seeds

When to Harvest for Medicinal Potency: Harvest leaves and stems under a waxing moon throughout the growing season. Harvest seeds when they are fully mature and dry to the touch.

HERBAL REMEDY TIP

A perfect example of "food as medicine," I love to toss leaves and stems into salads, soups, rice dishes, sauces and salsas. Additionally, coriander seeds are wonderful combined with cumin seeds for a warming spice blend.

Ashwagandha

Withania somnifera

Herbal Energetics: Warm/dry
Signatures: Soft, inviting

Widely regarded as a tremendously useful adaptogenic herb, ashwagandha is a profoundly effective herb for those suffering from chronic stress. Ashwagandha nourishes the adrenals, helping to restore a sense of calm and control for the chronically overburdened and overstressed, which through association, helps the immune system remain vital and strong. This herb is also a popular herb for reproductive complaints such as flagging libido, erectile dysfunction, low sperm count and irregular periods. Ashwagandha, paired with a healthy diet, exercise and stress reduction, can increase one's mental and physical stamina, while dialing back a heightened fight-or-flight response.

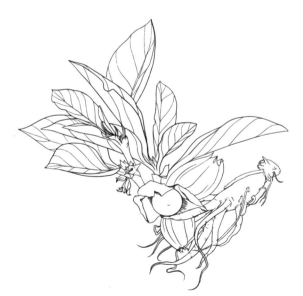

PLANT SNAPSHOT

Shrub
Zone: 6–12 (may act as an herbaceous perennial in zones 8 and below)
Growth Habit: Upright, somewhat woody shrub

GROWING THIS HEALING BOTANICAL

Light Requirements: Full sun

Garden Placement: This upright botanical can grow up to 4 feet (1.2 m) and should be placed near the back of a border or bed.

Soil Preference: Ashwagandha prefers dry, slightly sandy soils of low to moderate fertility.

When to Plant: Sow ashwagandha seeds indoors 10 to 12 weeks before last frost during an ascending moon. Transplant outdoors when the soil warms to approximately 65°F (18°C) during a waxing moon.

Best Growing Tips: Avoid planting near other nightshade family botanicals such as tomatoes, peppers, potatoes and eggplant to prevent spread of pests and disease.

Garden Companions: Plant ashwagandha near basil, oregano or dill to help deter unwanted pests.

HARVESTING THIS HERBAL ALLY

Parts Used: Roots, leaves (mildly medicinal), berries (edible but bitter)

When to Harvest for Medicinal Potency: Gently dig and prune roots in late fall under a descending moon. Fresh leaves can be gathered under a waxing moon throughout the growing season.

HERBAL REMEDY TIP

Prepare fresh, clean roots in a tincture (page 24) to restore one's vitality, while also committing to daily self-care including a healthy diet, exercise, outdoor time and stress reduction to support the entire adrenal system.

California Poppy

Eschscholzia californica

Herbal Energetics: Cool/dry
Signatures: Flexible, carefree

California poppy is heralded by herbalists for its calming effect on the central nervous system. This gentle botanical serves to soothe both the mind and body. California poppy is particularly useful for that "pins and needles" nerve pain but is also useful for addressing joint and muscle pain. It is a particularly wonderful choice for those who fail to have a satisfying night's sleep—while not overly sedative, it does dial down the sense of over stimulation, allowing for less sleep interruption. This herb is also beneficial for those who feel frenzied and easily distracted during the day.

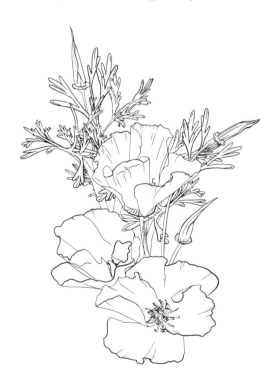

PLANT SNAPSHOT

Short-lived perennial
Zone: 8–10 (can be grown as an annual in cooler zones)
Growth Habit: Low growing, feathery

GROWING THIS HEALING BOTANICAL

Light Requirements: Full sun

Garden Placement: Plant California poppy near the front of borders where its wispy foliage and delicate flowers can be enjoyed.

Soil Preference: This botanical thrives in dry, rocky or sandy soils with low nutrient value.

When to Plant: Sow seeds directly into soil after all danger of frost has passed, under an ascending moon. California poppy does not appreciate root disturbance, so it is best to avoid transplant.

Best Growing Tips: California poppy is the perfect botanical to plant in areas that go untended, as it provides a wonderful blooming ground cover that will last all season while discouraging less desirable weeds.

Garden Companions: California poppy makes a stunning wild border with white Queen Anne's Lace, purple flowering verbenas and salvias.

HARVESTING THIS HERBAL ALLY

Parts Used: Leaves, flowers

When to Harvest for Medicinal Potency: Harvest leaves and flowers throughout the blooming season under a waxing moon.

HERBAL REMEDY TIP

As a tonic for the nervous system, I love a simple California poppy tincture (page 24). For increased sedative properties, combine with passionflower (page 86).

Chamomile (German)

Matricaria chamomilla/recutita

Herbal Energetics: Cool/dry
Signatures: Sunny, joyful and calm

One of the most widely embraced herbs by the general population, chamomile is well known as a popular remedy for inviting a restful slumber. Far from its only use, chamomile is a wonderful antispasmodic helping to reduce a persistent, irritating cough, stomach and intestinal cramping, uterine pain and irritability. In fact, chamomile may even provide relief from musculoskeletal and nerve pain. This herb is also a great wound treatment, cleansing and relieving inflammation from minor cuts, scrapes and burns.

PLANT SNAPSHOT
Perennial (short-lived but free-seeding)
Zone: 4–7
Growth Habit: Sprawling, open, low growing

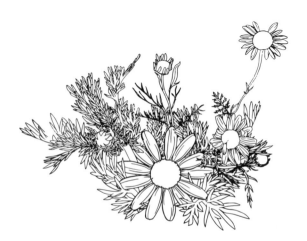

GROWING THIS HEALING BOTANICAL

Light Requirements: Full sun

Garden Placement: Chamomile is a great addition to any bed or border where one can easily rake their hands through the foliage to release the delicious apple-y aroma and gather the fresh blooms.

Soil Preference: This botanical likes moderately rich, loamy, well-drained soils and is fairly drought resistant in temperate climates once established.

When to Plant: Sow chamomile seeds indoors 6 to 8 weeks before last frost during an ascending moon; transplant outdoors when the plants reach about 4 inches (10 cm) tall, under a waxing moon.

Best Growing Tips: Chamomile can become quite sprawling and leggy if left untouched. Harvest flowers when they are fully opened and trim the plant back to 4 to 6 inches (10 to 15 cm) throughout the season to encourage compact growth and repeat blooms.

Garden Companions: Plant chamomile near basil, mint and roses to increase aromatic constituents or near brassica family vegetables to deter garden pests.

HARVESTING THIS HERBAL ALLY

Parts Used: Flowers

When to Harvest for Medicinal Potency: Gather flowers as soon as they are fully open, preferably during an ascending moon.

HERBAL REMEDY TIP

Perhaps it is "common use" but it is for a reason. My favorite way to enjoy chamomile is as a simple tea (page 22) for a soothing, calming act of daily self-care. We all deserve the powerful restorative action of sleep, and chamomile is a useful tool to achieve that!

Holy Basil/Tulsi

Ocimum tenuiflorum, sanctum, gratissimum

Herbal Energetics: Warm to cool (neutral)/dry
Signatures: Spiritual, creative, calming, grounding

As indicated by its common name, this fragrant member of the greater basil family (even culinary basil, O. basilicum, *can be similarly used for medicinal purposes), is an herb for grounding your being—calming your body and spirit. This adaptogenic herb is an excellent choice for reducing anxiety and sleeplessness. Additionally, holy basil can be used for a host of complaints such as digestive discomfort, pain and spasmodic conditions such as hiccups, menstrual cramping and coughing fits. Tulsi also helps the immune system by offering antimicrobial and detoxification benefits.*

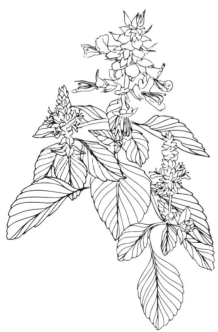

PLANT SNAPSHOT

Annual
Zone: 5–10
Growth Habit: Bushy, growing 2 to 4 feet (0.6 to 1.2 m) in size

GROWING THIS HEALING BOTANICAL

Light Requirements: Full sun

Garden Placement: Place holy basil toward the middle to the back of a bed or as a fragrant border. Full sun exposure will encourage flowering, so be sure to harvest regularly to encourage regrowth.

Soil Preference: Holy basil likes well-drained, loamy soils with moderate fertility. As it grows aggressively throughout the warmer season, it is helpful to compost and fertilize every 2 to 3 weeks.

When to Plant: Plant tulsi seeds indoors 4 to 6 weeks before the last expected frost or directly into the garden when the soil reaches 65 to 70°F (18 to 21°C), under a waxing moon. Plant seedlings outdoors when all danger of frost has passed, under a waning moon.

Best Growing Tips: Basil grows prolifically when given adequate water and fertility. Harvest the flowering tips as they emerge to ensure repeat growth.

Garden Companions: Plant near nightshades such as peppers, tomatoes and eggplant or near asparagus to attract ladybugs. Holy basil thrives next to borage and calendula as well.

HARVESTING THIS HERBAL ALLY

Parts Used: Leaves, flowering tips

When to Harvest for Medicinal Potency: Harvest leaves and flowering tips throughout the growing season under an ascending moon.

HERBAL REMEDY TIP

Fragrant and flavorful, holy basil is delicious as a tea or infusion (page 22). Enjoy the moment of making a tea combined with rose petals and chamomile for a transcendent olfactory experience.

Hops

Humulus lupulus

Herbal Energetics: Cool/dry
Signatures: Resilient

Best known as providing the bitter flavor in beer, hops are a likely and effective sedative herb. This botanical has an affinity for the central nervous system, acting to dial down an overactive state in the mind and body. Hops are perfect for those feeling overstimulated and unable to relax. This botanical helps one drift into a restful, restorative sleep. Additionally, hops relax the uterine and pelvic muscles, relieving painful cramping and promoting full bladder elimination.

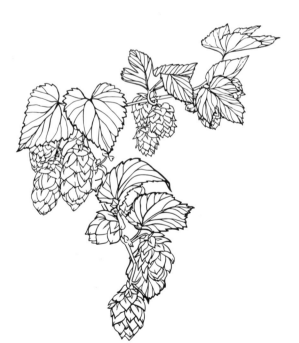

PLANT SNAPSHOT

Perennial
Zone: 5–9
Growth Habit: Trailing, clinging

GROWING THIS HEALING BOTANICAL

Light Requirements: Full sun

Garden Placement: Hops require support such as a very sturdy trellis or arbor for the "bines," the technical name for the vines.

Soil Preference: Hops prefer sandy, well-drained soils.

When to Plant: Commercial hops are propagated by root/rhizome division, but home gardeners may have more success cutting lengths of bines and burying them under sandy soil and loose mulch under a descending moon. Dig bines in mid-spring and cut 4- to 6-inch (10- to 15-cm) pieces and replant them during a waning moon to promote root growth.

Best Growing Tips: Due to the aggressive and fast-growing nature of hops, this botanical is ideally suited to growing on a sturdy pergola where you can enjoy the shade provided by the foliage and the harvest later in the season.

Garden Companions: The cones of hops are susceptible to insect infestation, so planting near chives, coriander and fennel can help prevent damage.

HARVESTING THIS HERBAL ALLY

Parts Used: Cones

When to Harvest for Medicinal Potency: Gather cones under an ascending moon in late summer or early fall.

HERBAL REMEDY TIP

A hops bath is truly one of the most relaxing experiences for the mind and body. Combine dried hops, rose petals (page 71) and lavender buds (page 110) in muslin drawstring bag, place in the bath water and soak away your troubles.

Lemon Balm

Melissa officinalis

Herbal Energetics: Cool/dry
Signatures: Sunny, bright

Soothing, calming, citrusy lemon balm is a wonderful herb for a variety of complaints ranging from loss of joy to insomnia, and it is even a potent remedy to fight viral issues. Providing gentle sedative and antispasmodic action, lemon balm is helpful for sleeplessness caused by mental and physical tension. Its uplifting nature bolsters spirits when the feeling of frenzied overwhelm sets in. It is an excellent remedy to address gas, bloating and colicky complaints. Additionally, as a potent antiviral, lemon balm is a chief herb for treating cold sores caused by the herpes virus.

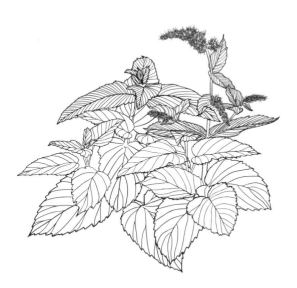

PLANT SNAPSHOT

Perennial
Zone: 4–9
Growth Habit: Spreading, upright

GROWING THIS HEALING BOTANICAL

Light Requirements: Full sun to partial shade

Garden Placement: Lemon balm begs to be touched to release its wonderful lemony fragrance, so plant this herb where it can be touched and harvested with ease.

Soil Preference: Adaptive to virtually any soil condition, lemon balm thrives best in moderately rich soil that is well draining.

When to Plant: Sow lemon balm seeds indoors about 8 to 10 weeks before the last frost during an ascending moon. Transplant seedlings after danger of frost has passed under a waning moon.

Best Growing Tips: Lemon balm will grow aggressively, so offer this botanical plenty of room to spread carefree. It is also a great herb to plant next to seating areas to repel biting insects.

Garden Companions: Lemon balm is a useful companion in the garden as it attracts pollinators, while warding off common garden pests.

HARVESTING THIS HERBAL ALLY

Parts Used: Leaves, flowering tips

When to Harvest for Medicinal Potency: Harvest lemon balm as the flowers just start to bloom during a waxing moon.

HERBAL REMEDY TIP

Lemon balm's citrusy flavor and aroma is somewhat delicate. As such I love to infuse it in water for a cooling sip on hot summer days to preserve its aromatics that are degraded by heat. To maximize its relaxing properties, create a tincture (page 24) with the leaves and flowering tips and take it in the evening to invite a restful night's sleep.

St. John's Wort

Hypericum perforatum

Herbal Energetics: Cool/dry
Signatures: Sunny, adaptive, willful

Perhaps best known as an antidepressant herb, St. John's wort offers a wide range of benefits for the entire nervous system. This botanical has a profound reputation for lessening the severity of mild to moderate depression and anxiety, particularly for those who display nervous irritability, tension and overall raw, exposed edginess. In the physical body, this herb soothes and calms nerve-inflamed fibers, making it a remedy to back/spinal pain, sciatica, shingles and nerve damage that deliver sharp pins and needles pain. St. John's wort also acts on tense spasmodic tissues of the digestive, reproductive, cardiovascular and musculoskeletal systems.

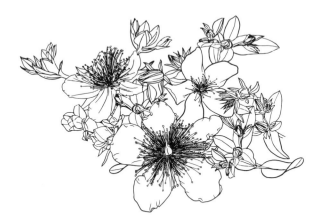

PLANT SNAPSHOT
Perennial
Zone: 5–9
Growth Habit: Upright

GROWING THIS HEALING BOTANICAL

Light Requirements: Full sun to partial shade

Garden Placement: Plant St. John's wort in masses in the midsection of a bed or border.

Soil Preference: St. John's wort thrives in relatively poor to moderate soils with excellent drainage.

When to Plant: Sow St. John's wort seeds directly in fall to allow for cold stratification.

Best Growing Tips: The most medicinally valuable species, *H. perforatum*, can appear somewhat weedy if planted sparsely, so plant in large groupings for a bolder effect. More ornamental species are quite striking and beautiful but little research exists regarding their medicinal use and potential for toxicity.

Garden Companions: Plant St. John's wort near yarrow and echinacea where they will enjoy similar conditions.

HARVESTING THIS HERBAL ALLY

Parts Used: Leaves, flowers

When to Harvest for Medicinal Potency: Harvest the fresh growing tips of St. John's wort as the flower starts to open, during a waxing moon.

HERBAL REMEDY TIP

Making a fresh St. John's wort tincture (page 24) is an act of inviting joy itself. The crushed leaves and flowers almost immediately emit a red dye that transforms a clear menstruum into the most inviting ruby elixir.

Oats

Avena sativa

Herbal Energetics: Cool/moist
Signatures: Flexible, graceful

Oats have served as a valuable food source and medicine for ages. This highly nutritious botanical is a functional food that is easily digestible when a person is feeling weak. Its mucilaginous characteristics offer gentle benefits to the digestive system and help bowel regularity. The milky sap from immature seeds is a touchstone herb for the central nervous system and mental health. Milky oats are a chief remedy for those who feel exhausted, frazzled and frayed around the edges.

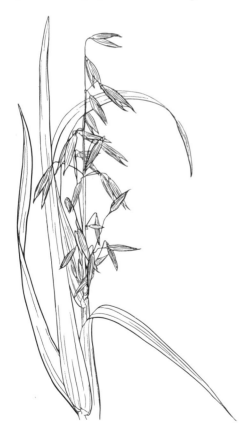

PLANT SNAPSHOT

Perennial
Zone: 3–9 (winter die-back will occur in colder regions of this spread)
Growth Habit: Upright, arching, slender

GROWING THIS HEALING BOTANICAL

Light Requirements: Full sun

Garden Placement: Oats are an outstanding cool season crop to grow in grassy areas and pastures but is also suitable for raised beds.

Soil Preference: Oats prefer well-drained, loamy soils of moderate fertility.

When to Plant: Broadcast oat seeds in early spring in a prepared planting bed, during an ascending moon. Cover with a thin layer of soil.

Best Growing Tips: While I chose to grow oats for the milky pods rather than as a cereal grain, I let much of the crop go to seed so that I can ensure regrowth year after year.

Garden Companions: Plant oats and clover together as a medicinal cover crop to reap the benefits personally while revitalizing the soil when the plant matter is composted.

HARVESTING THIS HERBAL ALLY

Parts Used: Milky seed pods, stem and mature seed (edible cereal grain)

When to Harvest for Medicinal Potency: Harvest milky seed pods when they exude a whitish sap when pressed between your fingers during a waxing moon.

HERBAL REMEDY TIP

Create a tincture (page 24) for nervous exhaustion by blending fresh milky oats with your chosen menstruum.

Chaste Tree/ Vitex

Vitex agnus-castus

Herbal Energetics: Warm/dry
Signatures: Ethereal, dignified

Chaste tree, also known as vitex or vitex berry, is a botanical strongly associated with female reproductive wellness. This herb supports a healthy hormonal balance and can elevate diminished progesterone levels. As such, herbalists lean on vitex for concerns of polycystic ovarian syndrome, premenstrual syndrome, tender and fibrous breast tissue and fertility. It is also considered a galactagogue and may help nursing mothers increase their milk supply. Additionally, it is a wonderful supportive treatment for hormonal acne. It may also be helpful for prostate concerns and low urine flow in men.

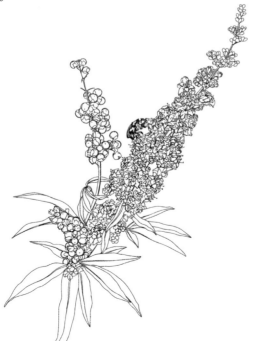

PLANT SNAPSHOT

Tree or shrub, depending on how it is pruned
Zone: 5–9 (may die back to the ground in zones 5–6 during harsh winters)
Growth Habit: Dense, vase-shaped

GROWING THIS HEALING BOTANICAL

Light Requirements: Full sun to partial shade

Garden Placement: The large bushy plant can grow upward of 20 feet (6 m) tall and quite wide, so give this stately botanical plenty of space.

Soil Preference: Chaste tree prefers light, well-drained soils. Low to modest soil fertility may help to keep its somewhat aggressive growth in check.

When to Plant: Plant established vitex specimens in the landscape during early spring under a waning moon.

Best Growing Tips: Chaste tree thrives in relatively poor conditions with minimal water or soil fertility, making it a great candidate for arid or xeriscaped gardens.

Garden Companions: Vitex's spicy and sage-like aroma is thought to deter a variety of garden pests. Plant near botanicals prone to insect damage.

HARVESTING THIS HERBAL ALLY

Parts Used: Berries

When to Harvest for Medicinal Potency: Harvest fruits as they start to turn a brown-black color and feel dry to the touch, usually late summer depending on climate.

HERBAL REMEDY TIP

I find vitex berries to be most effective when used as a tincture (page 24), especially during the luteinizing phase of the menstrual cycle, when it can be prepared as a tea with motherwort (page 90) and rose (page 71) for increased dosage.

Evening Primrose

Oenothera biennis

Herbal Energetics: Neutral/moist
Signatures: Expressive, statuesque

Evening primrose is a botanical often associated with women's health, but its benefits are far more expansive. This is an herbal remedy that acts on irritated and spasmodic tissues, making it an ideal botanical to address complaints of digestive discomfort, muscle spasms, coughing fits and uterine cramping. It is thought to soften the cervix and promote productive labor. Additionally, evening primrose nourishes the nervous system, making it a great ally for nerve pain, agitation, anxiety and addiction withdrawal.

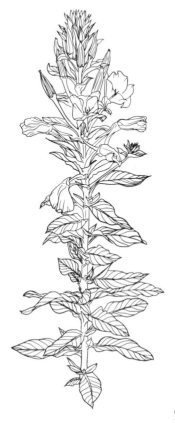

PLANT SNAPSHOT

Biennial
Zone: 5–8
Growth Habit: upright

GROWING THIS HEALING BOTANICAL

Light Requirements: Full sun to partial shade

Garden Placement: This striking botanical can grow to heights of 3 to 5 feet (0.9 to 1.5 m), so it is ideally planted near the back of ornamental borders.

Soil Preference: Evening primrose prefers slightly acidic, well-drained soils with ample water supply.

When to Plant: This herb needs cold stratification in order to germinate. As such, sow seeds directly into loose soil in fall under a waxing moon cycle.

Best Growing Tips: This lemony scented botanical blooms in late afternoon throughout the evening in shades of yellow (some species boasting whiter and rose-colored blooms). Plant evening primrose close to outdoor dining and seating where its blooms can be enjoyed.

Garden Companions: Evening primrose is a great attractor of pollinators and enjoys being planted near poppies.

HARVESTING THIS HERBAL ALLY

Parts Used: Leaves, flower, seeds, young roots

When to Harvest for Medicinal Potency: Gather leaves and flowers during a waxing moon throughout the summer. Young roots are best harvested in early fall under a descending moon. Seeds can be collected as they become dry to the touch.

HERBAL REMEDY TIP

Although evening primrose oil is readily available, albeit at a cost, I like to create a whole plant tincture (page 24) blended from plant material collected and tinctured during their ideal moon cycle.

Pumpkin

Cucurbita pepo

Herbal Energetics: Cool/damp
Signatures: Bountiful, generous

A hallmark symbol of the harvest season, pumpkin offers a host of medicinal benefits. Pumpkin seeds are highly valued for prostate complaints and urinary retention. Raw seeds are also consumed to dispel intestinal parasites and have a gentle laxative effect. Postpartum mothers may find that pumpkin seeds promote lactation and reduce fluid retention in the limbs. Pumpkin is a great potassium and magnesium source and as such, it supports cardiovascular health and helps maintain healthy blood pressure.

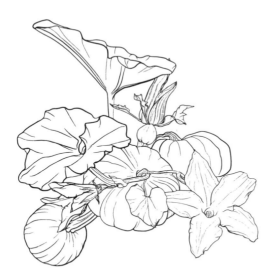

PLANT SNAPSHOT

Annual
Zone: 3–9
Growth Habit: Sprawling, vining

GROWING THIS HEALING BOTANICAL

Light Requirements: Full sun

Garden Placement: Plant pumpkin seeds where the meandering vines have room to roam.

Soil Preference: Pumpkins prefer rich, loamy well-drained soils.

When to Plant: Sow pumpkin seeds outdoors 2 to 4 weeks before last frost, or directly outdoors after frost danger has passed, during a waxing moon.

Best Growing Tips: Pumpkins are heavy feeders. Work compost into the soil to ensure a good pumpkin harvest.

Garden Companions: Pumpkins love to be planted with corn and pole beans, as well as melons, nasturtiums and oregano.

HARVESTING THIS HERBAL ALLY

Parts Used: Seeds, flesh (edible)

When to Harvest for Medicinal Potency: Harvest pumpkins in early fall during an ascending moon.

HERBAL REMEDY TIP

Save the seeds scooped from the pumpkin flesh. Roast some for a healthy snack while making a tincture (page 24) with the rest, blending the seeds with your chosen menstruum.

Red Clover

Trifolium pratense

Herbal Energetics: Cool/dry
Signatures: Flourishing, adaptive

Red clover is perhaps best known in the modern herbal pharmacopeia as a phytoestrogen used to calm menopausal complaints. This is an herb used to address concerns like hot flashes, mood swings, vaginal health and triglyceride levels in those who don't have hormone-sensitive conditions. It is a highly nutritive herb and is also considered a "blood purifier" and lymphatic mover. As such, this is an herb to make one feel lighter and brighter.

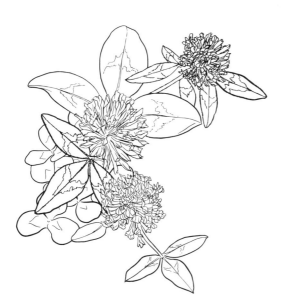

PLANT SNAPSHOT

Perennial
Zone: 3–9
Growth Habit: Low growing, mounding, spreading

GROWING THIS HEALING BOTANICAL

Light Requirements: Full sun

Garden Placement: Red clover is best planted in large swaths or naturalized to grassy areas.

Soil Preference: Due to its long taproot, red clover is capable of tolerating poor to moderate soil fertility and is adaptive to either dry or damp soil conditions.

When to Plant: Broadcast red clover seeds in late summer or early fall and allow seeds to overwinter.

Best Growing Tips: Red clover is an excellent herb to grow in grassy areas and open meadows where other herbs and grasses fail to thrive.

Garden Companions: Red clover is a legume and as such, it is friendly to botanicals like corn that enjoy the nitrogen-fixing abilities of this herb.

HARVESTING THIS HERBAL ALLY

Parts Used: Blossoms

When to Harvest for Medicinal Potency: Gather blossoms as they open, particularly under an ascending moon.

HERBAL REMEDY TIP

Red clover blossoms create a lightly flavored tea (page 22) when combined with chamomile (page 52) and spearmint (page 41) to deal with hot flashes and anxiety.

Raspberry

Rubus idaeus

Herbal Energetics: Cool/dry
Signatures: Bright, bold

A favorite summer fruit, the red raspberry leaves are a favored herbal medicine for lax tissues. Considered a uterine tonic, midwives and herbalists recommend this ally for mothers due to give birth. Additionally, it is suggested for excessive menstrual flow, cramping and vaginal discharge. Similarly, red raspberry leaves are an excellent remedy to help arrest diarrhea. Its tannic properties also offer relief from mouth sores and it may help dry up excessive sinus discharge.

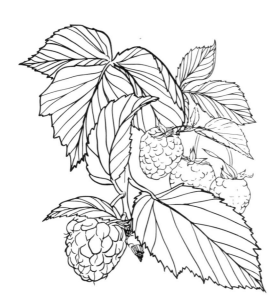

PLANT SNAPSHOT

Perennial
Zone: 3–9
Growth Habit: Vigorous, sprawling

GROWING THIS HEALING BOTANICAL

Light Requirements: Full sun

Garden Placement: Raspberries require sturdy support for ease of growth and harvest.

Soil Preference: Raspberries like rich, loamy soils that drain freely yet have some moisture-retentive properties.

When to Plant: Raspberries are most easily cultivated by division. Using a clean shovel, dig through established clumps and transplant them during a waning moon.

Best Growing Tips: Red raspberries bear fruit on the previous year's canes, so take special care when pruning to only remove dead canes in the spring.

Garden Companions: Plant allium family members like onions and garlic to help deter red raspberry pests.

HARVESTING THIS HERBAL ALLY

Parts Used: Leaves, fruit (edible)

When to Harvest for Medicinal Potency: Gather leaves early in the summer under an ascending moon.

HERBAL REMEDY TIP

Sipping a red raspberry leaf tea (page 22) is a restorative experience, with its floral, fruity aroma and flavor. Drink this as a daily tonic during the final weeks of pregnancy to promote productive labor.

Bee Balm

Monarda didyma, fistulosa

Herbal Energetics: Warm/dry
Signatures: Uplifting, encouraging

This aromatic, diffusive herb offers an abundance of medicinal uses, particularly for concerns of congestion and stagnation. The spicy nature of bee balm lends itself to complaints of lung congestion, wet, heavy cough and sinus pressure. It is also an excellent choice for addressing indigestion, cramping and a sense of a sour stomach. Due to its profoundly antiseptic qualities, bee balm can also be used to treat skin ulcers, sores and eruptive skin conditions. Its stimulating benefits can encourage perspiration and help reduce fever.

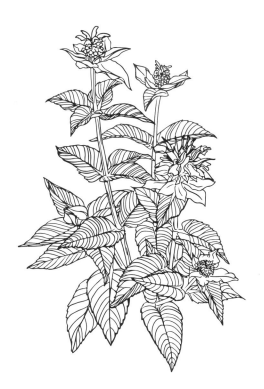

PLANT SNAPSHOT

Perennial
Zone: 3–9
Growth Habit: Upright, bushy

GROWING THIS HEALING BOTANICAL

Light Requirements: Full sun to light shade

Garden Placement: Most varieties grow to approximately 2 to 3 feet (0.6 to 0.9 m) tall so they are best planted near the midsection or back of a border.

Soil Preference: Bee balm tolerates a variety of soil conditions but does best when planted in well-drained soils of moderate fertility.

When to Plant: Plant seeds indoors about 8 weeks before the last frost or sow directly into the garden immediately after all danger of frost has passed under an ascending moon. Established plants can be easily divided, ideally under a waning moon to ensure good root development of the transplant.

Best Growing Tips: Gather blooming tips often throughout the growing season to ensure multiple sets of blooms.

Garden Companions: As a powerful attractor of pollinators, bee balm is a wonderful addition to the vegetable garden, berry patch or orchard.

HARVESTING THIS HERBAL ALLY

Parts Used: Leaves, flowers

When to Harvest for Medicinal Potency: Harvest the blooming tips and leaves throughout the growing season, under a waxing moon cycle.

HERBAL REMEDY TIP

Bee balm is a diffusive herb just meant for inhaling. Use this herb as a steam with lemon by tenting your head over a shallow bowl filled with the herb and water just off the boil. Inhale deeply to relax and relieve sinus congestion.

Honeysuckle

Lonicera japonica, periclymenu, sempervirens

Herbal Energetics: Cool/slightly damp
Signatures: Sweet, joyful

Heralded in traditional Chinese medicine for its affinity for the respiratory and digestive systems, honeysuckle is a somewhat underutilized botanical in Western herbalism. This slightly sweet, cooling herb calms inflamed respiratory tissues from illness and inhalation of heat and particulate matter. It may also relieve irritation caused by asthma, particularly of allergenic cause. It is also thought to have some antiviral benefits, possibly helping to prevent or minimize flu symptoms. Honeysuckle nourishes and promotes healthy digestive function, restoring vitality. This aromatic botanical is also thought to have a slight aphrodisiac benefit.

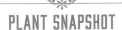

PLANT SNAPSHOT

Perennial
Zone: 5–9
Growth Habit: Twining, clinging vine

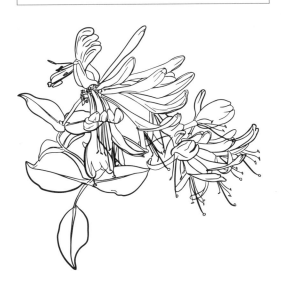

GROWING THIS HEALING BOTANICAL

Light Requirements: Full sun

Garden Placement: Plant honeysuckle where it can be supported by a trellis, post, fence or tree trunk/fallen branch.

Soil Preference: Honeysuckle prefers moist, loamy, well-drained soils of moderate fertility.

When to Plant: The fastest way to propagate honeysuckle is to take 6-inch (15-cm) cuttings from a well-established plant during a full moon. Remove all but the topmost leaves and pot in moist soil. Transplant honeysuckle when it is well established under a descending moon cycle.

Best Growing Tips: Although honeysuckle requires full sun for prolific blooms, its roots require cool, somewhat moist soil to thrive. Underplant this botanical with water-loving plants to shade and cool the soil.

Garden Companions: Shrubs such as roses, gooseberries and currants enjoy the same growing conditions as honeysuckle and provide cool shade for its roots.

HARVESTING THIS HERBAL ALLY

Parts Used: Flowers, berries (edible, except *L. sempervirens*, which are toxic)

When to Harvest for Medicinal Potency: Gather flowers just as they begin to bloom, early in the morning during an ascending moon, to enhance and preserve its aromatics.

HERBAL REMEDY TIP

Honeysuckle makes a soothing aromatic tea (page 22). It has a touch of perceived sweetness that can be enjoyed hot or cold. This is the perfect tea to sip while contemplating and appreciating the subtle beauty of life.

Hyssop

Hyssopus officinalis

Herbal Energetics: Warm/dry
Signatures: Showy, inviting

Hyssop is a notably diffusive herb both stimulating and relaxing to tissues and enhancing to the actions of adjunct herbs. The diffusive action of hyssop makes it an herb of merit for the respiratory and lymphatic systems. This is an herb to relieve congestion and tightness in the chest. It is a deeply "cleansing" botanical that can be used to encourage lymphatic drainage, helping one feel less stodgy, bloated and "full." Additionally, as a stimulating diaphoretic, hyssop can promote perspiration and assist in breaking a fever.

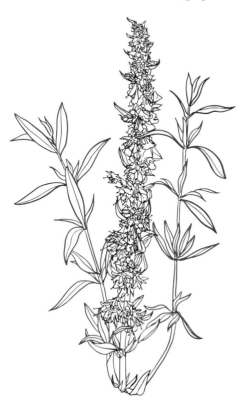

PLANT SNAPSHOT
Perennial
Zone: 4–9
Growth Habit: Upright, woody

GROWING THIS HEALING BOTANICAL

Light Requirements: Full sun

Garden Placement: Growing 18 to 24 inches (45 to 61 cm) tall and having a roaming nature, plant hyssop in the middle of a bed with plenty of room to spread.

Soil Preference: Hyssop prefer soils of moderate fertility and excellent drainage and can even thrive in poorer soils once it is well established.

When to Plant: Sow hyssop seeds 9 to 10 weeks before the last frost under a waxing moon. Transplant seedlings outdoors after all danger of frost has passed, during a descending moon.

Best Growing Tips: With its dark green foliage and beautiful whorls of lavender blooms and its ability to thrive in poor growing conditions, hyssop is a natural choice for planting in areas that are not frequently tended to.

Garden Companions: Plant hyssop near fellow diffusive herb bee balm in the vegetable garden where it will help repel flea beetles and lure cabbage moths away from brassica family crops.

HARVESTING THIS HERBAL ALLY

Parts Used: Leaves, flowers

When to Harvest for Medicinal Potency: Harvest the leaves and flowering tops throughout the blooming season just as the flowers begin to open under an ascending moon cycle.

HERBAL REMEDY TIP

The warm, minty, slightly woodsy aroma of hyssop is perfect for using in an herbal bath. Place hyssop leaves and/or flowers in a muslin drawstring bag and infuse in the bath water to relieve that stuck, stuffed, uncomfortable feeling associated with being ill and/or times of inactivity.

Milkweed/ Pleurisy Root

Asclepias species

Herbal Energetics: Cool/slightly moist
Signatures: Persistent, striking

As suggested by the common name, this botanical is considered a cardiovascular and respiratory tonic. Historically, milkweed has been used to treat pleurisy, which is painful inflammation of the chest wall. It is thought to help produce a strong, stable heartbeat in those in feeble states. As such, it is a wonderful herb to address mild asthmatic conditions. Pleurisy root offers healing potential to external concerns such as boils, wounds, warts and ringworm.

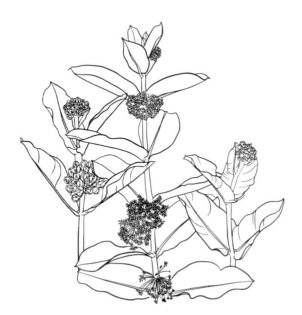

PLANT SNAPSHOT

Perennial
Zone: 4–9
Growth Habit: Upright

GROWING THIS HEALING BOTANICAL

Light Requirements: Full sun

Garden Placement: The many species of milkweed are perfectly adaptive to a variety of conditions, but it is most striking when left to naturalize in grassy meadow areas.

Soil Preference: The adaptive nature of pleurisy root provides species that are drought tolerant (whorled milkweed) to those that can withstand boggy conditions (swamp milkweed).

When to Plant: Sow milkweed seeds in early fall atop freshly turned over, clump-free soil. Alternatively, they can be successfully propagated from established plants by taking 4- to 6-inch (10- to 15-cm) cuttings and placing them in water during a waxing moon cycle until the roots are well developed.

Best Growing Tips: Choose a species of milkweed well adapted to your soil conditions and watch it flourish year after year.

Garden Companions: Plant pleurisy root near echinacea in drier areas or boneset in boggier locations. A great attractor of pollinators, this botanical can be added to orchards and berry patches.

HARVESTING THIS HERBAL ALLY

Parts Used: Roots

When to Harvest for Medicinal Potency: Gather roots from established milkweed patches in late summer under a descending moon.

HERBAL REMEDY TIP

Pleurisy root is a profoundly effective remedy when there is painful tightness in the ribs and dry cough. Try taking a tincture (page 24) three to four times while these symptoms persist, paying close attention to your body's need to rest and recuperate.

Mustard

Sinapis alba (yellow/white), Brassica nigra (brown)

Herbal Energetics: Warm/dry
Signatures: Pungent, spicy, bold

Far from just a popular condiment, mustard is an outstanding, if under-utilized, medicinal herb. Served as a functional food, this botanical opens airways, clears stodgy congestion and stimulates a visceral warmth. It is an excellent adjunct treatment for cold, damp conditions of the chest when there is a deep, wet cough that rattles one's frame. Mustard offers action against bacterial and fungal concerns. Its incredible warming benefits also make it an appropriate choice for arthritic joints affected by cold.

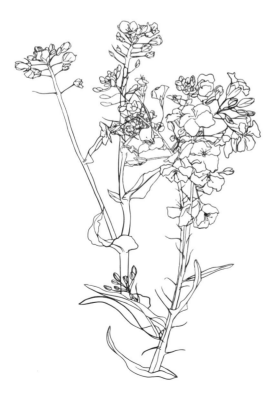

PLANT SNAPSHOT
Annual
Zone: 6–11
Growth Habit: Aggressive, bold

GROWING THIS HEALING BOTANICAL

Light Requirements: Full sun

Garden Placement: Mustard will flourish and grow to approximately 3 feet (0.9 m) tall in most conditions. As such, give it ample space and adequate airflow to prevent disease.

Soil Preference: Mustard prefers well-drained soils of moderate fertility.

When to Plant: Mustard prefers cooler weather. As such, sow mustard seeds in fall for an early spring crop.

Best Growing Tips: Mustard is a crop that will outcompete many other botanicals, so give it space to reach its potential without affecting other nearby plants.

Garden Companions: Mustard grows well in the vicinity of onions, garlic and other sturdy herbs such as rosemary and yarrow.

HARVESTING THIS HERBAL ALLY

Parts Used: Leaves (edible), seeds

When to Harvest for Medicinal Potency: Gather leaves for meals during cool spring and early summer mornings during an ascending moon. Seeds can be harvested as they become dry to the touch, mid- to late summer.

HERBAL REMEDY TIP

A classic remedy for deep chest colds and discomfort is to apply a "plaster" of dried mustard powder and water layered over muslin and applied to the skin for 10 to 20 minutes (remove sooner if there is a burning sensation).

Gentian

Gentiana species

Herbal Energetics: Cool/dry
Signatures: Resilient

Gentian is an intensely astringent herb with an array of medicinal uses for concerns of excessive discharge and eruptive skin conditions. While not an herb used widely in North American herbal medicine practices, gentian has been used by European, Middle Eastern and Asian practitioners for centuries to address complaints of digestive discomfort, bloating, heartburn, urinary retention and excessive menstrual flow. Its detoxifying nature lends itself to promoting liver and kidney function. Topically, gentian helps clear acne and soothe redness and irritation associated with seborrheic dermatitis, eczema, psoriasis and even poison oak/ivy.

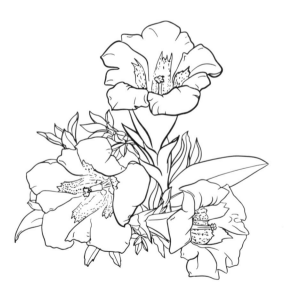

PLANT SNAPSHOT

Perennial
Zone: 4–7
Growth Habit: Mounding

GROWING THIS HEALING BOTANICAL

Light Requirements: Full sun to partial shade (especially in hotter growing areas)

Garden Placement: Growing approximately 2 feet (0.6 m) in height, gentian is best grown in the middle of borders and beds, as well as being well suited to containers.

Soil Preference: Gentian prefers cool, well-drained, sandy or rocky soils.

When to Plant: Needing cold for better germination, sow seeds in early fall under a waning moon, covering lightly with soil and keeping moist until the damp weather sets in.

Best Growing Tips: Gentian is considered an "alpine" plant. As such, it is well adapted to the harsher growing conditions and coolness of mountainous regions.

Garden Companions: The rare true-blue flowers of gentian (although certain species offer white or yellow blooms) compliment the orange and yellow shades of calendula.

HARVESTING THIS HERBAL ALLY

Parts Used: Root

When to Harvest for Medicinal Potency: Harvest roots in late summer or early fall as the blooms start to fade under a descending moon.

HERBAL REMEDY TIP

Gentian is a wonderful skin treatment to promote clear, firm skin. Create a cold infusion (page 23) using witch hazel and apply to the skin as a toning mist or by soaking cotton discs.

Jamaican Dogwood

Piscidia piscipula, erythrina

Herbal Energetics: Warm/dry
Signatures: Gentle, sheltering

PLANT SNAPSHOT

Tree or large shrub, depending on early-stage pruning
Zone: 10–13
Growth Habit: Erect

Not commonly used in the western herbal landscape, Jamaican dogwood is a native herb worth exploring for its profound benefits to the central nervous and musculoskeletal systems. Herbalists have used this herb to address unsettling nerve pain, sciatica and arthritic conditions. Jamaican dogwood is also known to soothe smooth muscle tissue, making it an excellent remedy for digestive and uterine cramping. As a stimulating diaphoretic, the botanical can induce perspiration and reduce a fever.

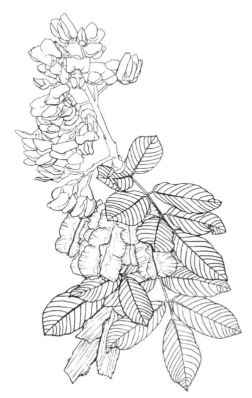

GROWING THIS HEALING BOTANICAL

Light Requirements: Full sun to light shade

Garden Placement: The medium-sized tree can grow quite large under the right conditions, so give it ample space to reach its potential.

Soil Preference: Jamaican dogwood thrives in dry, slightly sandy, relatively poor soils.

When to Plant: Scarify Jamaican dogwood seeds by nicking or sanding part of the outer seed coating and soak seeds for 6 hours or overnight. Sow seeds in pots during an ascending moon, and place them in a warm sunny spot to germinate. Transplant the seedlings outdoors once they are well established, during a waning moon.

Best Growing Tips: Jamaican dogwood can withstand some brackish or saltwater exposure. As such, it is an excellent choice for seaside plantings in tropical and subtropical regions.

Garden Companions: Underplant Jamaican dogwood with subtropical and tropical plants that may tolerate its shade, such as citronella and lemongrass.

HARVESTING THIS HERBAL ALLY

Parts Used: Bark

When to Harvest for Medicinal Potency: Harvest the pliable bark by carefully and thoughtfully pruning small limbs and stripping the bark with a sharp knife during an ascending moon.

HERBAL REMEDY TIP

Jamaican dogwood is best tinctured (page 24) and taken when pain is persistent. It is thought to be an excellent choice for a physically traumatic event, allowing the body to rest and recover while relieving acute pain.

Oak

Quercus species

Herbal Energetics: Cool/dry
Signatures: Stately, unwavering

The majestic oak is not a terribly common botanical in the modern herbal pharmacopeia, but nonetheless, is a powerful ally in the apothecary. Due to its incredibly high tannin content, oak is an astringent remedy of lax and oozy conditions of the skin such as acne, blisters, burns, oozing wounds and various seborrheic conditions of the skin. A mist or compress of cooled oak infusion can be especially soothing to weeping sunburns. Internally, oak may help with excessive mucus in the stomach and arrest diarrhea.

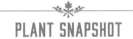

PLANT SNAPSHOT

Tree
Zone: 3–10 depending on species
Growth Habit: Upright, full

GROWING THIS HEALING BOTANICAL

Light Requirements: Full sun

Garden Placement: Oaks should be planted where they can grow to their full height potential and where one may desire shade in the future.

Soil Preference: Oaks prefer rich, well-drained soil.

When to Plant: Acorns can be planted in spring during an ascending moon. Place larger established trees into the landscape during a waning moon.

Best Growing Tips: Growing oaks is an exercise in patience that pays off for future generations. If you have an oak in your landscape, appreciate its placement.

Garden Companions: The great canopy of oak creates ample shadow for shade-loving herbs such as lady's mantle and bugleweed.

HARVESTING THIS HERBAL ALLY

Parts Used: Inner bark, acorns (edible)

When to Harvest for Medicinal Potency: Harvest the inner bark from fallen or cut wood as it presents itself or scrape from pruned branches during an ascending moon.

HERBAL REMEDY TIP

Create a cooled decoction (page 23) of oak mixed with aloe to make a soothing remedy for sunburns when applied as a mist or compress.

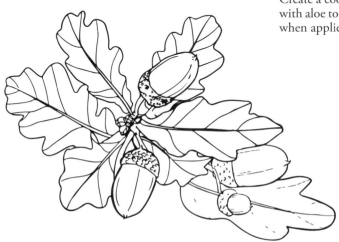

Rose

Rosa species

Herbal Energetics: Cool/dry
Signatures: Elegant, stately, strong

From the formal tea roses to the feral and carefree wild species, roses are a mainstay of the garden and the apothecary. Roses are perfectly suited to a variety of irritable conditions. The botanical is ideal for calming anxious and flustered mental states and can gently uplift those experiencing blue states. The petals of rose are at once astringent and emollient—both acting to tone and moisturize the skin. Rosehips are bursting with vitamin C; as such, they are a powerful antioxidant and a foremost ally in the fight against cold and flu. Additionally, rose can tone red, bleeding gums, soothe oral sores and relieve a sore and scratchy throat.

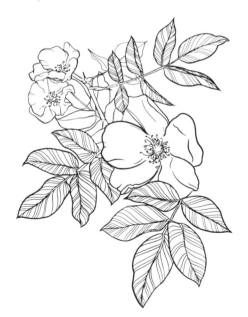

PLANT SNAPSHOT
Shrub
Zone: 3–11
Growth Habit: Upright to vining

GROWING THIS HEALING BOTANICAL

Light Requirements: Full sun

Garden Placement: Roses are often grown as a foundation shrub or standard (grafted and pruned to a tree shape), so place the rose as a focal point in the landscape. Some varieties are bred to climb and are best grown on sturdy arbors or walls.

Soil Preference: Roses like loamy, well-drained soils with ample fertility.

When to Plant: Plant bare root roses early to mid-spring during a descending moon.

Best Growing Tips: Roses need airflow to prevent humidity-related diseases like black spot and powdery mildew. Water at soil level and prune to keep an open, airy canopy.

Garden Companions: Plant yarrow near roses as it is supposed to increase the aromatic constituents of rose.

HARVESTING THIS HERBAL ALLY

Parts Used: Leaves, flowers, rosehips

When to Harvest for Medicinal Potency: Gather leaves and petals (leaving the capsule to form a hip) throughout the summer during an ascending moon, early in the morning. Rosehips can be harvested in fall when they are bright red (or orange depending on the variety), under a waxing moon.

HERBAL REMEDY TIP

Rose petal tea (page 22) with chamomile (page 52) is the perfect way to reverse the ravages of a frustrating day. Sip while practicing measured, calm breathing, perhaps while soaking in a petal strewn bath to release tension.

Arnica

Arnica montana

Herbal Energetics: Warm/dry
Signatures: Courage, strength

Arnica is a premier first aid treatment for bruising, sprains, strains, shin splints and even broken or dislocated bones. Arnica acts to clear damaged cells and speed the recovery process of many blunt force and exertion-related activities. Arnica gently warms and rushes fresh blood flow to cold, stiff and frozen joints to restore flexibility and mobility. This herb is also recommended for chilblain (painful transition from cold to warm in the fingers and toes) and is regarded well for nerve pain. Note that arnica is recommended for external use only.

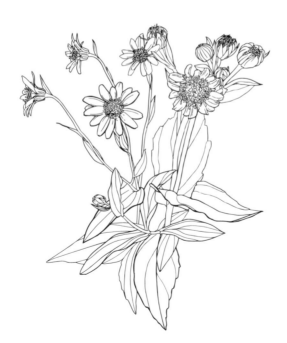

PLANT SNAPSHOT

Perennial
Zone: 4–9
Growth Habit: Low growing, clumping

GROWING THIS HEALING BOTANICAL

Light Requirements: Full sun or partial shade if grown in hotter climates

Garden Placement: Plant arnica in rock gardens and alkaline areas where other plants struggle, toward the front of a border or bed.

Soil Preference: Arnica thrives in shallow, sandy or rocky, well-drained and even slightly alkaline soils.

When to Plant: Sow arnica seeds directly into prepared soil and cover lightly with damp sand.

Best Growing Tips: While arnica prefers dry conditions, it does require irrigation. Water when the top 2 inches (5 cm) of soil feels dry.

Garden Companions: Arnica thrives in similar "alpine" or mountainous conditions as gentian.

HARVESTING THIS HERBAL ALLY

Parts Used: Leaves, flowers

When to Harvest for Medicinal Potency: Harvest leaves and flowers throughout the blooming season during an ascending moon.

HERBAL REMEDY TIP

Arnica produces a lovely orange infused oil (page 27) that can be used as a soothing massage oil or transformed into a salve (page 27) for targeted treatment of injuries or unbroken skin.

Calendula

Calendula officinalis

Herbal Energetics: Cool/neutral
Signatures: Sunny, uplifting, generous

Perhaps one of the most useful herbs in the apothecary, calendula offers a tremendous bevy of medicinal uses. Known extensively for its ability to heal and close cuts and abrasions, calendula is a star botanical for wound treatment. Additionally, applied topically, it serves to cool inflamed skin, while its astringent and simultaneously emollient properties help skin remain firm, soft textured and supple. Internally, calendula is an excellent choice for dry, scratchy throats, especially those irritated by hot, dry weather and particulate matter in the air. This herb is also capable of soothing the stomach of heartburn, ulcers and digestive complaints as it repairs tissues damaged by inflammation. As a powerful lymphatic, calendula is also beneficial for relieving stagnation in the lymph clusters in the neck, underarm/breast area and groin.

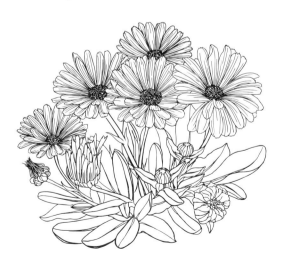

PLANT SNAPSHOT

Annual
Zone: 2–11 (perennial in zones 9–11)
Growth Habit: Sprawling, somewhat mounding

GROWING THIS HEALING BOTANICAL

Light Requirements: Full sun or light shade

Garden Placement: Plant calendula close to the front of borders and in any area that you want to be filled in year after year as this botanical is a *generous* reseeder.

Soil Preference: This herb grows best in average or even poor soil fertility but does need adequate moisture.

When to Plant: Due to its somewhat frost hardy nature, calendula can be sown outdoors in early spring under a waxing moon cycle.

Best Growing Tips: Calendula will bloom from late spring until the weather cools considerably in late fall. It is a prime candidate for successive seed sowing in spring or allowing some flowers to seed throughout the growing season.

Garden Companions: This sunny flower is a perfect garden ally for the vegetable patch or more fragile plants like roses that are susceptible to aphids.

HARVESTING THIS HERBAL ALLY

Parts Used: Flowers

When to Harvest for Medicinal Potency: Harvest buds just as the buds begin to open during an ascending moon.

HERBAL REMEDY TIP

There are so many wonderful uses for this herb, but chief among them is creating a golden-hued healing salve (page 27) for minor wounds and abrasions using calendula-infused oil (page 27).

Helichrysum/ Immortale

Helichrysum italicum

Herbal Energetics: Warm/dry
Signatures: Open, radiant, glowing

Praised for its tremendous healing benefits, fragrant helichrysum (sometimes referred to as curry plant) is a powerful yet gentle herb for the home apothecary. As a vulnerary herb, helichrysum offers great healing potential for wounds, promoting closure, reducing scar tissue formation and clearing bruises and irritating scabs. Perhaps a reference to its other commonly used name, immortale, this herb also promotes a radiant firm complexion due to its exceptional antioxidant potential. Internally, this herb helps soothe inflamed bronchial tissue and promote proper digestive action.

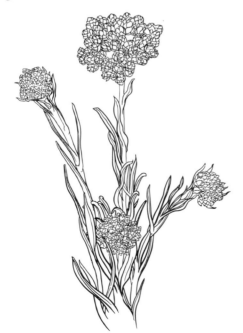

PLANT SNAPSHOT

Perennial
Zone: 5–11 (may be grown as an annual in cooler zones)
Growth Habit: Open, airy mounds

GROWING THIS HEALING BOTANICAL

Light Requirements: Full sun

Garden Placement: Place helichrysum near the front to middle of the border where the petite vibrant yellow blooms and silvery fragrant foliage can be enjoyed.

Soil Preference: Helichrysum prefers light, even slightly sandy soils that drain freely.

When to Plant: Sow seeds indoors 3 to 4 weeks before the last frost under an ascending moon.

Best Growing Tips: Plant helichrysum in masses so that its delicate flowers and foliage don't get lost among bolder plantings.

Garden Companions: This herb thrives in the same conditions as lavender and rosemary.

HARVESTING THIS HERBAL ALLY

Parts Used: Leaves, flowers

When to Harvest for Medicinal Potency: Harvest flowering tips throughout the blooming season under an ascending moon.

HERBAL REMEDY TIP

Helichrysum dries beautifully, making it a perfect herb for infusing in oil (page 27) for a moisturizing, occlusive facial treatment or as a base for healing salves (page 27).

Lamb's Ear

Stachys byzantina

Herbal Energetics: Cool/moist
Signatures: Soft, caring

This fuzzy botanical is known as nature's bandage. Its naturally absorbent properties, along with its antiseptic, antimicrobial and anti-inflammatory benefits make it an excellent treatment for wound care. It is also a soothing treatment for itchy, bloodshot eyes and styes. Taken internally, it is thought to help heal esophageal erosion, digestive heat, diarrhea and even mild internal bleeding. It can also soothe a dry itchy throat and reduce a fever.

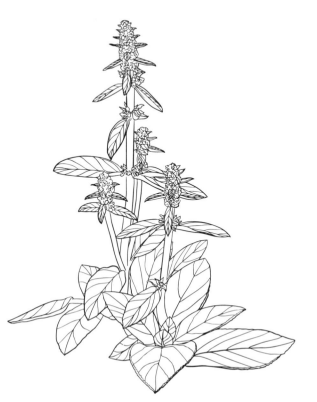

PLANT SNAPSHOT

Perennial
Zone: 4–8
Growth Habit: Erect, dense, upright spikes

GROWING THIS HEALING BOTANICAL

Light Requirements: Full sun

Garden Placement: With its fuzzy, silvery foliage, lamb's ear accentuates darker foliage herbs planted toward the middle or back of a border. It is also a fun botanical to plant along walking paths, as its soft foliage invites curious fingers for touch.

Soil Preference: Lamb's ear thrives in loamy, well-drained soils of moderate fertility.

When to Plant: Lamb's ear is most successfully propagated by division. Using a clean, sharp shovel or trowel, divide existing clumps and plant the new divisions under a descending moon.

Best Growing Tips: This botanical is susceptible to mildew and humidity-related disease, so it is imperative to avoid overhead watering to prevent soaking the thick, downy leaves.

Garden Companions: As a natural deer deterrent, plant lamb's ear near berries, roses and other botanicals prone to grazing.

HARVESTING THIS HERBAL ALLY

Parts Used: Leaves

When to Harvest for Medicinal Potency: Gather leaves from established plants during an ascending moon cycle.

HERBAL REMEDY TIP

Lambs ear is the perfect quick remedy for addressing small nicks and cuts while working in the garden. Just pluck a leaf and apply it directly to the skin!

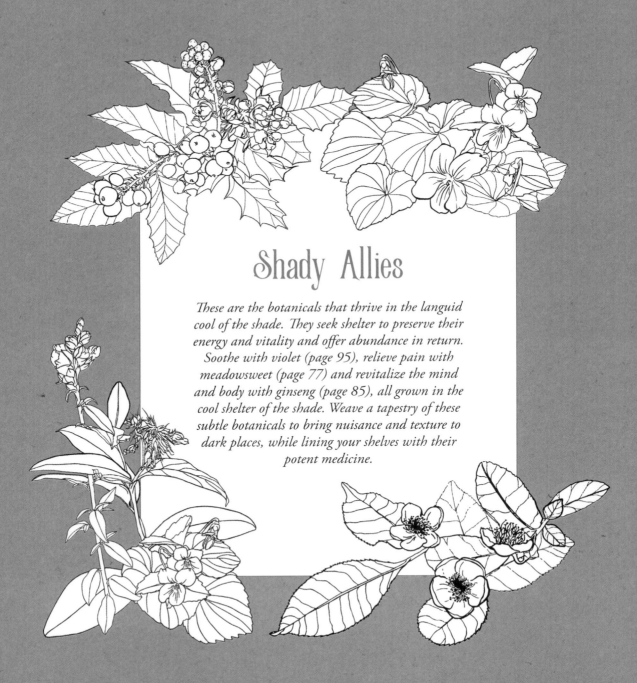

Shady Allies

These are the botanicals that thrive in the languid cool of the shade. They seek shelter to preserve their energy and vitality and offer abundance in return. Soothe with violet (page 95), relieve pain with meadowsweet (page 77) and revitalize the mind and body with ginseng (page 85), all grown in the cool shelter of the shade. Weave a tapestry of these subtle botanicals to bring nuisance and texture to dark places, while lining your shelves with their potent medicine.

Meadowsweet

Filipendula ulmaria

Herbal Energetics: Cool/dry
Signatures: Radiant, beckoning

Meadowsweet is the ideal herb for those of a hot constitution with stomach complaints. Meadowsweet is ideal for those who suffer from poor digestive action (that too-full feeling), nausea, heartburn and indigestion. It is an excellent remedy for gastric ulcer pain and gastric reflux. Meadowsweet promotes perspiration and can help relieve a fever. Additionally, meadowsweet is a good herb to address bleeding, irritated, inflamed gums and mouth sores.

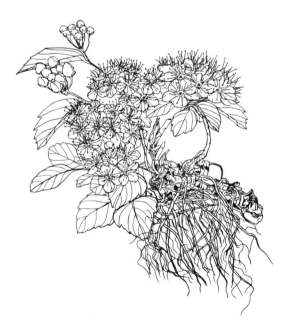

PLANT SNAPSHOT

Perennial
Zone: 3–8
Growth Habit: Arching, open

GROWING THIS HEALING BOTANICAL

Light Requirements: Partial or dappled shade

Garden Placement: Meadowsweet is perfect for woodland borders where its height and fragrant light blooms beckon.

Soil Preference: This botanical thrives in rich well-drained, humus-rich soils.

When to Plant: Meadowsweet is most easily propagated from cuttings. During a descending moon, remove the lower leaves from 4- to 6-inch (10- to 15-cm) trimming and place it in water until roots are well established. Transplant outdoors during a waning moon.

Best Growing Tips: Meadowsweet will wither and brown without frequent watering, so although it doesn't like wet feet, place it where it can be adequately irrigated.

Garden Companions: As a deer deterrent, meadowsweet can help protect more attractive crops from grazing.

HARVESTING THIS HERBAL ALLY

Parts Used: Leaves, flowers

When to Harvest for Medicinal Potency: Gather leaves and flowers during an ascending moon.

HERBAL REMEDY TIP

Meadowsweet tea (page 22) is the perfect after-meal beverage to improve digestion and soothe indigestion, especially for those who tend to be hot and experience flushing after eating.

Camellia

Camellia sinensis

Herbal Energetics: Cool/dry
Signatures: Shiny, bold, dramatic, strong

Better known as the plant that produces black, green, white and oolong teas, camellias are a true medicinal plant. Camellia is highly tannic and helps to control excessive mucus in the digestive system. As such, camellia is an excellent remedy for diarrhea. Applied externally, camellia reduces the redness and weeping from a blistering sunburn. As a gentle stimulant, camellia may temporarily increase energy, reduce anxiety and help with weight loss. Offering antioxidant action, this herb also promotes cellular repair.

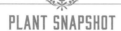

PLANT SNAPSHOT

Evergreen shrub
Zone: 7–9
Growth Habit: Bushy, full, upright, woody

GROWING THIS HEALING BOTANICAL

Light Requirements: Partial shade with morning sun

Garden Placement: Plant camellias where they can receive morning sun but are shaded from harsh afternoon rays, with plenty of space to reach its 10- to 15-foot (3- to 4.5-m) height and substantial spread.

Soil Preference: Camellias prefer moderate rich, slightly acidic, well-drained, loamy soils.

When to Plant: Most easily propagated by cuttings, trim camellia shoots in early spring during a descending moon. Remove the bottom leaves of a 4- to 6-inch (10- to 15-cm) trimming and set it in water until roots form. Transplant to soil when the roots are well established under a waning moon.

Best Growing Tips: Camellia produces dense foliage, making it an excellent hedge botanical.

Garden Companions: Camellias thrive with other acid-tolerant botanicals like ground elder, ferns, firs and beth root.

HARVESTING THIS HERBAL ALLY

Parts Used: Leaves

When to Harvest for Medicinal Potency: Gather leaves during late spring and early summer under a waxing moon.

HERBAL REMEDY TIP

Camellia sinensis is the tea (page 22) we are all familiar with. Choose between the varieties (black, green, white and oolong) that are created by different drying and curing techniques based on flavor, mouthfeel and personal preference.

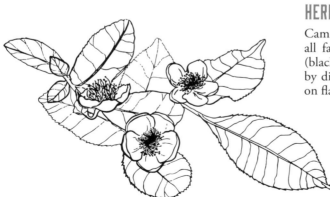

Sassafras

Sassafras albidum, officinale

Herbal Energetics: Warm/dry
Signatures: Intense, alluring

Somewhat out of favor in the modern herbal pharmacopeia, sassafras is part of traditional medicine of the indigenous peoples of North America. This intensely spicy herb was once used as a remedy for diarrhea and as an antidote to foul water poisoning. It has been used to address complaints of sore, achy joints while improving circulation. As a potent warming herb, sassafras can be used to promote perspiration for those experiencing lingering fevers that are plagued with cold and shivers.

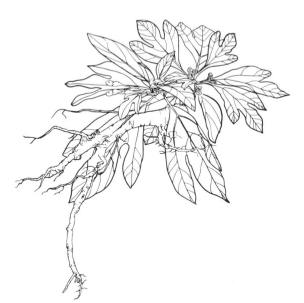

PLANT SNAPSHOT

Shrub or tree depending on pruning techniques
Zone: 4–9
Growth Habit: Upright spreading

GROWING THIS HEALING BOTANICAL

Light Requirements: Partial shade

Garden Placement: Sassafras is best suited to the edges of woodland gardens where it can receive dappled sun.

Soil Preference: Sassafras thrives best in loamy soils with a light, sandy texture.

When to Plant: Sassafras is most easily propagated from root cuttings. Dig up a small 6- to 8-inch (15- to 20-cm) lateral root and transplant it to its desired spot during a waning moon.

Best Growing Tips: Since the medicinal portion of this botanical is the bark, encourage branching low in the bush by pruning down the topmost branches.

Garden Companions: Sassafras is considered somewhat allelopathic, meaning they seem to discourage undergrowth. While hardly a "friendly" garden companion, it discourages undesirable undergrowth in areas that one prefers to be clear of vegetation.

HARVESTING THIS HERBAL ALLY

Parts Used: Bark, leaves (edible)

When to Harvest for Medicinal Potency: Harvest bark and leaves throughout the growing season under an ascending moon.

HERBAL REMEDY TIP

Create a decoction (page 23) using sassafras bark, cinnamon and ginger for a spicy drink to invigorate digestion and warm you from the inside out. Avoid alcohol-based remedies such as tinctures due to potential toxicity.

Astragalus

Astragalus membranaceus

Herbal Energetics: Warm/damp
Signatures: Understated, embracing

Long used in traditional Chinese medicine, astragalus is now heralded as an adaptogenic herb with incredible immune-modulating activity. Considered a preventative health tonic, astragalus has profound anti-inflammatory and antimicrobial properties making an outstanding herb during the cold and flu season. Astragalus helps the body adapt to physical, mental and emotional stressors and has profound antioxidant activity, which may prevent cellular damage. Additionally, astragalus acts as a gentle diuretic, helping to relieve bladder discomfort and edema.

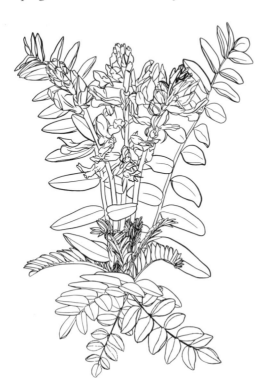

PLANT SNAPSHOT

Perennial
Zone: 6–11
Growth Habit: Mounding, fernlike

GROWING THIS HEALING BOTANICAL

Light Requirements: Partial shade (can tolerate full sun in colder climates)

Garden Placement: Astragalus boasts softs foliage that resembles of combination of pea and fern, with yellow or purple flowering spikes. Growing 1 to 3 feet (0.3 to 0.9 m) tall, the astragalus is well suited to a mixed woodland garden.

Soil Preference: Astragalus prefers soils slightly acidic to neutral, loamy, well-drained soils of moderate fertility.

When to Plant: This medicinal herb germinates best after a controlled cold stratification period. Refrigerate dampened seeds for at least 3 weeks, then sow indoors 8 to 10 weeks before last frost during a waxing moon. Transplant well-established seedlings after danger of frost has passed under a descending moon.

Best Growing Tips: Put astragalus where it will be easy to dig and harvest the roots. When harvesting, leave some roots to grow the next season.

Garden Companions: As a member of the greater pea family, astragalus benefits heavier feeders like snapdragons and other shade-tolerant botanicals.

HARVESTING THIS HERBAL ALLY

Parts Used: Roots

When to Harvest for Medicinal Potency: Harvest roots from 2- to 3-year-old and older plants during a waning moon.

HERBAL REMEDY TIP

While astragalus is a great remedy as a tincture (page 24), an infusion (page 22) will help to reap the benefits of its polysaccharide content. Simmer it in a broth with mushrooms and herbs to create a healing soup.

Oregon Grape

Mahonia aquifolium

Herbal Energetics: Cool/dry
Signatures: Striking, defensive

Brimming with berberine, Oregon grape is one of nature's most outstanding antibiotics. Oregon grape is particularly good for upper respiratory infections, particularly with postnasal drip that produces a persistent, irritable cough and stomach discomfort. Additionally, this herb is ideally suited for diarrhea caused by bacteria, such as in food poisoning. Oregon grape also supports liver health, reduces inflammation and can soothe red, oozy skin conditions.

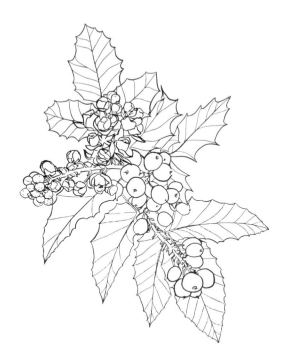

PLANT SNAPSHOT
Shrub
Zone: 5–9
Growth Habit: Evergreen, upright, holly-like

GROWING THIS HEALING BOTANICAL

Light Requirements: Full shade to partial sun

Garden Placement: Place Oregon grape near the back or borders and beds where it can grow to its height potential of 3 to 10 feet (0.9 to 3 m) high, with a spread of up to 5 feet (1.5 m).

Soil Preference: Oregon grape prefers humus-y fertile, well-draining, deep soils to accommodate its extensive root system.

When to Plant: The botanical is most easily propagated by taking cuttings. During a waning moon, place 4- to 6-inch (10- to 15-cm) cuttings with the lower leaves removed in water until roots develop. Transplant cuttings when roots are well established during a descending moon cycle.

Best Growing Tips: The tips of Oregon grape are quite sharp, and one should avoid planting them near travel paths. By the same token, due to the sharp leaves, this a popular botanical to place under windows to deter burglars from accessing a home.

Garden Companions: This botanical thrives in similar conditions as huckleberry and blueberry, as well as many other acid-loving plants. It may also deter grazing animals from crops such as lettuces and ornamentals like hostas.

HARVESTING THIS HERBAL ALLY

Parts Used: Inner bark, roots and berries (edible)

When to Harvest for Medicinal Potency: Harvest roots and inner bark from lower branches during a descending moon.

HERBAL REMEDY TIP

Oregon grape is an excellent tincture (page 24) to have on hand when one suspects sinus infection.

Spilanthes (Toothache Plant)

Acmella oleracea

Herbal Energetics: Warm/neutral
Signatures: Diminutive, surprising

Spilanthes is widely regarded as an herb for oral health. The "electric" flavor sensation produces a numbing effect perfect for addressing acute toothaches, as well as providing pain relief for TMJ sufferers. This botanical promotes the salivary response helping those with dry mouth complaints and assisting with the first stages of digestion. It is also an excellent herb for fighting mouth thrush complaints and gum inflammation. Additionally, spilanthes is a powerful immune system stimulant, making it a great remedy for the cold and flu season.

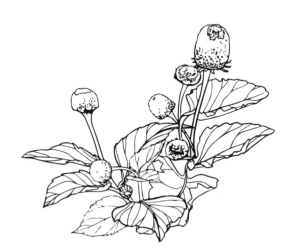

PLANT SNAPSHOT
Annual
Zone: 10–12 (grown as an annual in cooler regions)
Growth Habit: Low growing, mounding

GROWING THIS HEALING BOTANICAL

Light Requirements: Partial shade to full sun (where some protection from afternoon rays can be had)

Garden Placement: Place spilanthes near the front of a border and plant in masses for a more striking effect from the diminutive flowers.

Soil Preference: Spilanthes prefers relatively rich, loamy, somewhat moisture-retentive soils.

When to Plant: Sow spilanthes seeds 8 to 10 weeks before last frost under a waxing moon.

Best Growing Tips: Spilanthes likes warm soil and frequent watering. As such, this plant thrives near buildings that radiate warmth to the plant. Harvest flowers frequently to promote rebloom.

Garden Companions: Spilanthes thrives in similar conditions as strawberries and makes a striking combination.

HARVESTING THIS HERBAL ALLY

Parts Used: Flower

When to Harvest for Medicinal Potency: Gather flowers throughout the growing season during an ascending moon.

HERBAL REMEDY TIP

Although fresh spilanthes can be chewed straight from the garden for toothache complaints, tincture flowers (page 24) for use when oral complaints strike throughout the year.

Ground Elder

Aegopodium podagraria

Herbal Energetics: Cool/dry
Signatures: Sheltering, embracing

Unrelated to elderberry (Sambucus)*, ground elder has its own great medicinal value by way of its benefits to the urinary tract. As a profound diuretic, it is an excellent choice for those experiencing edema and swelling of the joints. Also known as goutwort, this botanical has long been used by those suffering from painful gout symptoms. It is also a mild sedative, producing a calming effect and helping to induce a restful sleep. Additionally, applied externally, its astringent properties may assist with hemorrhoids and varicose veins.*

PLANT SNAPSHOT
Perennial
Zone: 4–9
Growth Habit: Creeping, dense ground cover

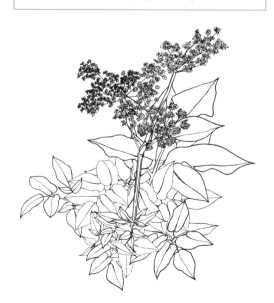

GROWING THIS HEALING BOTANICAL

Light Requirements: Partial shade (shelter from harsh afternoon rays)

Garden Placement: Plant ground elder where it has plenty of room to spread and cover ground. It is ideally suited to northern exposures when not shaded as it is prone to leaf scorch.

Soil Preference: Ground elder is adaptive to a variety of soil conditions, but thrives in slightly acidic and damp soils.

When to Plant: Although it can be grown from seed, ground elder is most easily propagated from division. As spring shoots emerge, dig and separate clumps and transplant them during a descending moon.

Best Growing Tips: Ground elder is particularly hardy, even considered invasive. It is resistant to chemical sprays and can thrive where herbicides have previously been applied (wait a couple years before harvesting for medicinal use) and can be used for erosion control.

Garden Companions: Ground elder thrives near camellias and black cohosh.

HARVESTING THIS HERBAL ALLY

Parts Used: Leaves, flowers, seeds

When to Harvest for Medicinal Potency: Gather leaves and flowers throughout the growing season during an ascending moon. Seeds can be harvested when they become dry to the touch in mid-summer, under a waxing moon.

HERBAL REMEDY TIP

The leaves of ground elder are a suitable salad green and can impart flavors reminiscent of celery and fennel, making this a great functional food. Drinking tea of ground elder (page 22), one can benefit from its diuretic properties.

Hydrangea
Hydrangea aborescens

Herbal Energetics: Cool/dry
Signatures: Dramatic, generous, persevering

The wild hydrangea, sibling of showier landscaping cultivars, is a valuable herb for the home apothecary with its profound affinity for the urinary tract. Hydrangea is a gentle diuretic and antispasmodic and may assist in the passing of kidney stones. It can also relieve a sense of persistent bladder fullness and mild cystitis. Hydrangea is also for specific prostatic concerns, such as benign hyperplasia. It may also assist with the digestion of fats and gallbladder irritation.

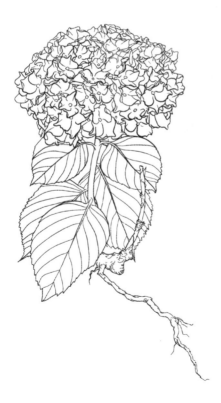

Shrub
Zone: 3–9
Growth Habit: Woody, open

GROWING THIS HEALING BOTANICAL

Light Requirements: Partial to full shade

Garden Placement: Under the right growing conditions, hydrangeas can grow to a spread of 3 to 6 feet (0.9 to 1.8 m) tall and wide and even larger given time. As such, give them plenty of space to grow.

Soil Preference: This botanical prefers cool loamy soils of moderate fertility.

When to Plant: Hydrangeas are most easily propagated by cuttings. During a waning moon, take a 4- to 6-inch (10- to 15-cm) cutting, strip all but the topmost leaves and place the cuttings in water. Transplant when the roots are well established under a descending moon.

Best Growing Tips: Hydrangeas are prone to scorching and sensitive to drought conditions, so plant where they can receive irrigation during hot summer.

Garden Companions: Underplant hydrangeas with violets to keep the soil cool and moist during the summer months.

HARVESTING THIS HERBAL ALLY

Parts Used: Roots

When to Harvest for Medicinal Potency: It is difficult to avoid killing a plant when harvesting roots, but careful root trimming can be achieved by pulling back the soil and trimming the roots with clean shears, under a waning moon, and recovering with soil.

HERBAL REMEDY TIP

Like many root-based remedies, hydrangea lends itself well to tinctures (page 24). Take a dropperful before a meal to promote digestion or if plagued by kidney discomfort.

Ginseng

Panax ginseng (Asian), quinquefolius (American)

Herbal Energetics: Warm/damp

Signatures: Persistent, strong, understated

Both Asian and American ginseng are prized as heralded health tonics. Ginseng is considered a powerful adaptogenic herb, increasing energy and stamina and boosting overall vitality. Ginseng supports mental clarity and cognition and can elevate one's "can do" attitude. This herb is also thought to support sexual health, improving a flagging libido. Rich in antioxidants, ginseng protects cells from damage and illness. This botanical also helps maintain healthy blood sugars.

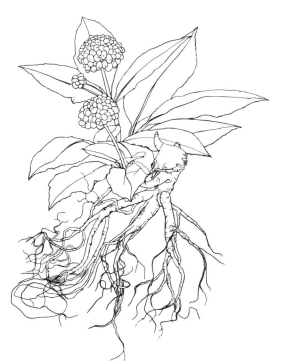

PLANT SNAPSHOT

Perennial

Zone: 3–7

Growth Habit: Low growing, open ground cover

GROWING THIS HEALING BOTANICAL

Light Requirements: Full shade to partial shade

Garden Placement: Plant ginseng under the canopy of large trees with other woodland botanicals where it can slowly spread and naturalize.

Soil Preference: Ginseng needs cool, moist, humus-rich soils with high nutrient value to thrive.

When to Plant: Sow ginseng seeds in fall or early winter to allow for cold stratification and the breakdown of the seed's outer layer.

Best Growing Tips: Ginseng requires commitment and takes 3 to 4 years before the roots are ready to harvest.

Garden Companions: Plant ginseng under the canopy of deciduous trees such as maple and cottonwood/poplars to mimic its native habitat.

HARVESTING THIS HERBAL ALLY

Parts Used: Roots

When to Harvest for Medicinal Potency: Gather roots from well-established ginseng plantings in early fall during a waning moon.

HERBAL REMEDY TIP

While ginseng is a superb daily tonic when taken in tincture form (page 24), great benefits can be experienced when combined with a diet rich in plant nutrients to support the body's natural detoxification process.

Passionflower

Passiflora incarnata

Herbal Energetics: Cool/dry
Signatures: Spiritual, exotic

The fantastical-looking passionflower is a superb tonic for the nervous system. Passionflower dials down the volume on a busy mind, allowing those with nervous exhaustion to fall into a restful sleep. For those prone to anxiety and burnout, this herb can help one relax and focus. As an antispasmodic, passionflower can relieve menstrual cramps, heart palpitations and restless legs. It can help normalize blood pressure and it's effective against nerve pain.

PLANT SNAPSHOT

Perennial
Zone: 5–9
Growth Habit: Vining

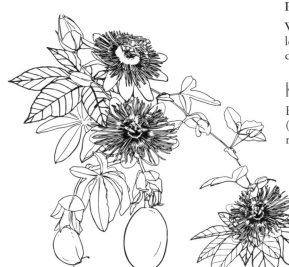

GROWING THIS HEALING BOTANICAL

Light Requirements: Partial shade (can tolerate full sun if given afternoon protection)

Garden Placement: Grow passionflower on a trellis or arbor to support its sprawling vines.

Soil Preference: Passionflower likes rich, slightly acidic and slightly moisture-retentive soils.

When to Plant: Scarify passionflower seeds slightly with sandpaper or the edge of a knife, then soak them in water for 1 to 2 days, discarding any floating seeds. Sow seeds in damp potting mix during a waxing moon and place them in plastic to create a humid environment to encourage germination. Transplant established seedlings under a descending moon.

Best Growing Tips: Passionflower leaves often turn yellow when in less-than-optimal conditions, particularly when underwatered or grown in a cold spot, so be willing to make adjustments as needed.

Garden Companions: Plant passionflower near onions, garlic or chives to deter pests and near berry patches to attract pollinators.

HARVESTING THIS HERBAL ALLY

Parts Used: Leaves, flowers

When to Harvest for Medicinal Potency: Harvest leaves and flowers throughout the growing season during a waxing moon.

HERBAL REMEDY TIP

Brew a passionflower tea (page 22) with rose (page 71) and chamomile (page 52) to induce a restful slumber without grogginess upon waking.

Sweet Woodruff

Galium odoratum

Herbal Energetics: Cool/dry
Signatures: Blanketing, unassuming, protective

Sweet woodruff is a gentle herb offering quiet, sedative properties. It is a great choice for those experiencing physical and mental tension, and for those who feel nervous and overwhelmed. It is a remedy for menopausal complaints, as well as menstrual cramping. It encourages digestion and heartens an appetite, especially for those with anxious stomachs. Sweet woodruff can encourage a steady, regular heartbeat and gently tone the urinary tract.

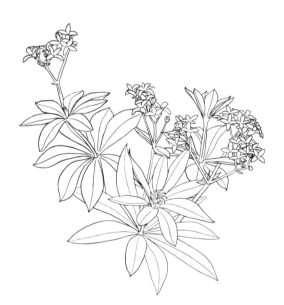

PLANT SNAPSHOT

Perennial
Zone: 3–8
Growth Habit: Spreading, ground cover

GROWING THIS HEALING BOTANICAL

Light Requirements: Partial to full shade

Garden Placement: Sweet woodruff thrives in dappled shade in the front of woodland borders and along footpaths.

Soil Preference: This highly adaptive herb grows well in a variety of soil conditions and is a good candidate for dry shade.

When to Plant: Sweet woodruff is most easily propagated by division. Divide established beds in early spring as new growth emerges and transplant during a waning moon.

Best Growing Tips: Sweet woodruff does not like hot, humid conditions and is great for naturalizing shaded areas where it can outcompete less desirable botanicals. Cut back after the first flush of flowering to encourage growth and rebloom.

Garden Companions: One of the few botanicals resistant to juglone, sweet woodruff is the perfect ground cover for planting under black walnut trees.

HARVESTING THIS HERBAL ALLY

Parts Used: Leaves, flowers

When to Harvest for Medicinal Potency: Harvest the flowering tips of this botanical during an ascending moon.

HERBAL REMEDY TIP

Dried sweet woodruff has a hay-honey scent and makes a lovely tea (page 22) for bringing calm. May wine is a celebratory drink of white wine infused with dried sweet woodruff and strawberries.

Beth Root

Trillium grandiflorum, erectum, pendulum

Herbal Energetics: Cool/dry
Signatures: Gentle, nodding, alluring

Beth root is an astringent herbal ally used to arrest all manner of discharges. Beth root has been used for a variety of menstrual complaints including excessive flow. It is also used to encourage productive labor during childbirth and help prevent hemorrhage. Beth root is effective for treating diarrhea and mucus in the digestive system. Applied externally, the herb can be used to tone weepy wounds and minor burns.

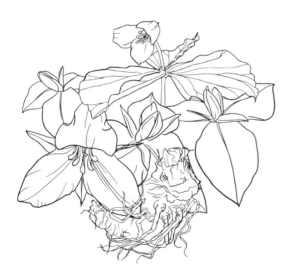

PLANT SNAPSHOT

Perennial
Zone: 4–9
Growth Habit: Low growing, erect, drooping blooms

GROWING THIS HEALING BOTANICAL

Light Requirements: Full shade

Garden Placement: Beth root is a stunning addition to the shadiest areas of woodland gardens with its nodding white or burgundy blooms.

Soil Preference: This botanical prefers nutrient rich, slightly acidic, humus-y soils that are moisture-retentive.

When to Plant: Beth root is most easily propagated by division. Separate existing clumps in early spring, transplanting divisions during a waning moon.

Best Growing Tips: Beth root is a welcome addition to the woodland landscape, where crawling insects like ants aid in naturalizing the understory by carrying the slow-to-germinate seeds over the soil.

Garden Companions: Beth root grows well in the shady protection and acidic soils of fir forests.

HARVESTING THIS HERBAL ALLY

Parts Used: Roots

When to Harvest for Medicinal Potency: Lift beth roots in early fall during a waning moon.

HERBAL REMEDY TIP

Tincture (page 24) fresh beth root and take as a menstrual self-care routine to relieve cycle complaints.

False Unicorn

Chamaelirium luteum

Herbal Energetics: Cool/dry
Signatures: Otherworldly, ethereal

This rare botanical has been associated with women's health and fertility. False unicorn is thought to help regulate hormones and support regular menstrual cycles by restoring estrogen balance. It tones and nourishes the uterus and cervix. It is valued when there are concerns of threatened miscarriage and may help elevate HCG levels. False unicorn may also assist in the treatment of polycystic ovarian syndrome and is a mild diuretic for bladder complaints.

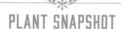

PLANT SNAPSHOT

Perennial
Zone: 5–8
Growth Habit: Mounding with tall flowering spikes

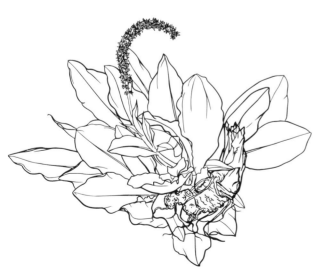

GROWING THIS HEALING BOTANICAL

Light Requirements: Full shade

Garden Placement: This slow growing botanical is ideal for the deep shade of woodland landscapes.

Soil Preference: False unicorn prefers cool, humus-y, moisture-retentive soils that are high in organic matter.

When to Plant: This herb is best suited to rhizome division in early spring. Gently lift the root system and divide rhizomes with visible "eyes" and transplant them during a waning moon.

Best Growing Tips: Nearing endangered status as a wild plant, it is imperative that herbalists seek out cultivated false unicorn for the apothecary. This heavy feeding botanical requires thoughtful mulching and nutrients to be successful.

Garden Companions: False unicorn grows best in the dense shade of conifers and as such is an excellent understory plant.

HARVESTING THIS HERBAL ALLY

Parts Used: Roots

When to Harvest for Medicinal Potency: Gather roots in early fall under a descending moon from a well-established planting. Note that false unicorn rarely returns from leftover root and rhizome material, so be thoughtful in gathering this plant.

HERBAL REMEDY TIP

Due to its rarity, this herb is best tinctured (page 24) for maximum extraction and potency and should be used sparingly to respect its delicate nature.

Motherwort

Leonurus cardiaca

Herbal Energetics: Warm/dry
Signatures: Bold, strong

Both the common and scientific names of this botanical suggest its use. Motherwort is often used to support women's health as it tones the uterus, reduces menstrual and menopausal complaints, and may help stimulate strong, productive contractions in childbirth. It is also an herb that has a profound affinity for the nervous system, reducing anxiety and helping those who are shy and retreating to take up their own space. Motherwort may also improve cardiac function by supporting the heart, maintaining healthy blood pressure and reducing spasmodic chest palpitations.

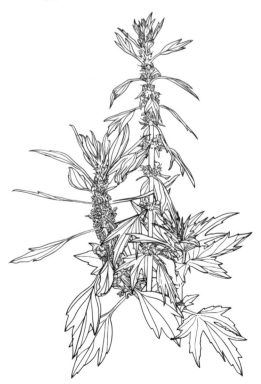

PLANT SNAPSHOT
Perennial
Zone: 4–8
Growth Habit: Towering, upright

GROWING THIS HEALING BOTANICAL

Light Requirements: Part or dappled shade

Garden Placement: Place motherwort near the back of shady borders, where it can achieve its height and not obstruct the view of more diminutive plants.

Soil Preference: Motherwort grows well in neglected soils where water supply is ample.

When to Plant: Scatter motherwort seeds in chosen areas in early fall to allow for cold stratification.

Best Growing Tips: Motherwort takes a while to establish. As such, give it 2 years to reach its height and flowering potential.

Garden Companions: Underplant motherwort with violets and self-heal where they can enjoy the additional shade of this botanical while keeping soils cool and moist.

HARVESTING THIS HERBAL ALLY

Parts Used: Leaves, flowers

When to Harvest for Medicinal Potency: Gather leaves and flowers throughout the growing season under a waxing moon.

HERBAL REMEDY TIP

Motherwort is ideal for acute spasmodic complaints such as cramping and anxiety attacks accompanied by a fluttery feeling in the chest. Therefore, I prefer to recommend this herb in tincture form (page 24).

Comfrey

Symphytum officinale

Herbal Energetics: Cool/moist
Signatures: Flexible, yielding

Sometimes colloquially known as knitbone, comfrey has a long and storied history of "knitting" damaged tissues together. Comfrey is an herb to use when tendons, ligaments, bones and skin are injured. This herb is perfect for superficial wounds when no sign of infection is present (not recommended when infection is suspected, since it is so efficient in bringing tissue closure). Internally, this is an herb to address concerns of heartburn and esophageal burning. Additionally, comfrey is a premier herb for concerns of varicose veins and hemorrhoids.

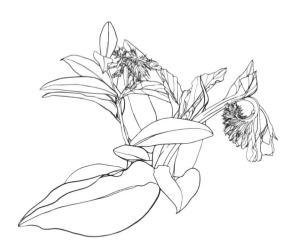

PLANT SNAPSHOT

Perennial/Annual/tree/shrub
Zone: 4–9
Growth Habit: Mounding

GROWING THIS HEALING BOTANICAL

Light Requirements: Partial shade to full sun (prefers afternoon shade)

Garden Placement: Comfrey will outcompete many other botanicals, so place it in areas where it has room to grow and where other plants fail to take hold.

Soil Preference: Comfrey prefers well-drained soils but is well adapted to a variety of soil conditions.

When to Plant: Sow seeds directly about 2 to 3 weeks before the last frost during an ascending moon.

Best Growing Tips: Comfrey is a botanical well suited to a variety of conditions; as such, plant it freely where other plants fail to thrive.

Garden Companions: Comfrey is a mainstay of permaculture guild planting. This is an outstanding botanical to underplant in orchards and where one seeks to provide increased soil fertility such as in small orchards.

HARVESTING THIS HERBAL ALLY

Parts Used: Roots, leaves

When to Harvest for Medicinal Potency: Gather leaves throughout the growing season during a waxing moon. Dig up roots in early fall under a waning moon.

HERBAL REMEDY TIP

Pack damp comfrey leaves onto sprains and strains and cover with a light fabric such as muslin to reduce pain and discomfort and assist the healing process.

Jewelweed

Impatiens capensis

Herbal Energetics: Cool/neutral
Signatures: Gentle, delicate

It is not often that a poison and an antidote can be found side by side, but that is just the case with jewelweed and a common forest-dwelling irritant. Jewelweed thrives in the same environment as poison oak, ivy and sumac and is largely considered one of the most effective remedies against the intense itching and red, scaly rash produced by the offending botanicals. It is also effective to treat sprains, strains and bruising. Most modern herbalists suggest this for topical use only due to its high calcium oxalate content.

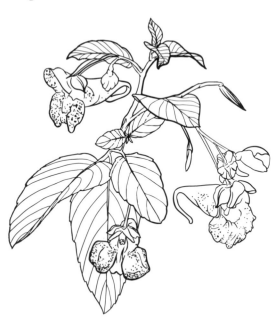

PLANT SNAPSHOT

Free-seeding annual
Zone: 2–11
Growth Habit: Arching, open

GROWING THIS HEALING BOTANICAL

Light Requirements: Full shade

Garden Placement: Place jewelweed in dense or dappled shade where it has room to reseed itself freely.

Soil Preference: Jewelweed prefers fertile, humus-rich moisture-retentive soils.

When to Plant: Gather fresh seeds from existing plants and scatter on freshly raked-over soils during an ascending moon.

Best Growing Tips: The stems of jewelweed are fragile and prone to breakage, so plant this botanical away from high traffic areas and shelter from harsh winds.

Garden Companions: Plant in the woodland understory of maples, poplars and alders, where it can be shaded and protected.

HARVESTING THIS HERBAL ALLY

Parts Used: Stems, leaves, flowers

When to Harvest for Medicinal Potency: Gather the aerial parts of jewelweed under an ascending moon.

HERBAL REMEDY TIP

Crush the stems, leaves and flowers of jewelweed and place in ice cube trays; fill with water and freeze for a quick and easy poultice to place on an erupting rash.

Snapdragon

Antirrhinum majus

Herbal Energetics: Cool/dry
Signatures: Joyful

Much better known for its colorful addition to cottage gardens, containers and flowerbeds, snapdragons have medicinal virtues to match their beauty. Snapdragons offer great astringent properties, making them an excellent remedy for weepy conditions such as watery eyes, bleeding gums and acne. Additionally, this botanical may be used to address hemorrhoids, varicose veins and blisters. These properties extend to the treatment of mild burns, speeding pain relief and reducing inflammation upon application.

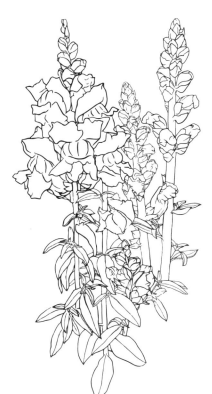

PLANT SNAPSHOT

Perennial
Zone: 7–11 (grown as an annual in cooler zones)
Growth Habit: Upright, dense

GROWING THIS HEALING BOTANICAL

Light Requirements: Partial shade (can tolerate full sun if given protection from late afternoon rays)

Garden Placement: Snapdragons are best placed near the middle or back of a flower border.

Soil Preference: These botanicals are light feeders and prefer well-drained soils and frequent watering.

When to Plant: Start snapdragons seeds indoors 8 to 10 weeks before last frost during a waxing moon. Transplant outdoors after the danger of frost has passed during a descending moon.

Best Growing Tips: Shear spent flower spikes throughout the growing season to encourage prolific reblooming.

Garden Companions: As a powerful attractor of pollinators, place snapdragons near crops like tomatoes, peppers and eggplant.

HARVESTING THIS HERBAL ALLY

Parts Used: Flowers, leaves

When to Harvest for Medicinal Potency: Gather the flowers and foliage just as the flowers open throughout the growing season during a waxing moon.

HERBAL REMEDY TIP

Snapdragons are a perfect quick garden first aid when made into a poultice and applied to minor burns!

Solomon's Seal

Polygonatum biflorum

Herbal Energetics: Cool/damp
Signatures: Graceful

Known for its affinity for connective tissue and the musculoskeletal systems, Solomon's seal is a prized botanical for aches and pains. This is the ideal remedy for those plagued by stiffness in the ligaments and tendons from injury, overuse, illness and aging. Solomon's seal may ease pain and inflammation in arthritic joints. Internally, it is a soothing demulcent for the respiratory and digestive systems, while also acting as an antispasmodic to reduce cramping. As a gentle diuretic, it helps to flush the kidneys and reduce water retention.

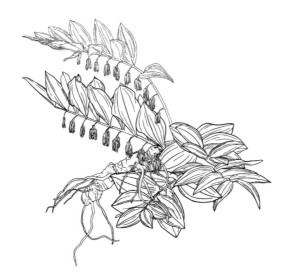

PLANT SNAPSHOT

Perennial
Zone: 3–9
Growth Habit: Upright, arching

GROWING THIS HEALING BOTANICAL

Light Requirements: Partial to full shade

Garden Placement: The tall arching stems and flowering shoots are a dramatic backdrop when placed near the back of a shady bed.

Soil Preference: Solomon's seal thrives in rich, cool, somewhat moist soils but is adaptive to dry shade conditions.

When to Plant: Divide clumps of rhizomes as shoots arise in spring and transplant them during a waxing moon.

Best Growing Tips: This is a somewhat slow-growing botanical that is being over-harvested in the wild landscape. As such, it is imperative and ethical to only harvest it from cultivated and home-grown plots.

Garden Companions: Solomon's seal grows beautifully among lungwort and wild ginger.

HARVESTING THIS HERBAL ALLY

Parts Used: Rhizomes and young shoots (avoid older shoots, leaves and berries as they are mildly toxic)

When to Harvest for Medicinal Potency: Harvest young, fleshy rhizomes during early to midsummer during a descending moon.

HERBAL REMEDY TIP

Tincture fresh rhizomes (page 24) and use in daily self-care practice with stretching exercises to maintain mobility and flexibility.

Violet

Viola species (particularly *odorata*)

Herbal Energetics: Cool/damp
Signatures: Gentle, soft, comforting

Violets are at their glory in the cool, moist days of spring, and perhaps this is an appropriate suggestion of their medicinal uses. Violets are a cooling, demulcent herb that relieves red, inflamed, hot, dry and cracked tissues. As such, violets lend themselves as remedy for tight dry coughs, itchy skin, bloodshot dry eyes, dehydrated ashy skin, minor burns, calluses, irritated genitals and hemorrhoids. Violet is also a widely regarded lymphatic, helping to encourage the flow of fluids especially about the neck, underarm/breast and groin. Additionally, violet can be used to address hot, dry conditions of the digestive systems such as heartburn and constipation.

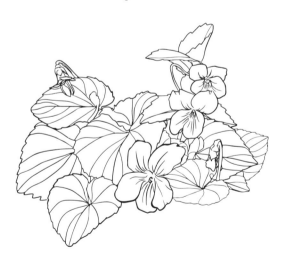

PLANT SNAPSHOT

Perennial
Zone: 3–9
Growth Habit: Spreading ground cover

GROWING THIS HEALING BOTANICAL

Light Requirements: Partial to full shade

Garden Placement: This relatively carefree, low-growing botanical is great in woodland settings and showier species such as *V. tricolor* are show-stoppers in shady containers.

Soil Preference: Violets prefer cool, rich, somewhat moist, loamy soils.

When to Plant: Violets are most easily propagated by cutting. Remove a leaf with a few inches of stem and place it in water until roots form. Transplant under a waning moon.

Best Growing Tips: Violets thrive in cool spring conditions and will often fade in summer heat. Plant violets in areas that remain consistently cool such as the north side of structures and well shaded areas.

Garden Companions: Violets thrive in similar conditions as wild ginger and sweet woodruff but are also a lovely addition to grassy areas where grass may be sparse and prone to moss due to shade.

HARVESTING THIS HERBAL ALLY

Parts Used: Leaves, flowers

When to Harvest for Medicinal Potency: Gather flowers and leaves in early spring as blooming commences during a waxing moon.

HERBAL REMEDY TIP

The greatest nutritive and demulcent benefits of violet are acquired in water base solutions for internal purposes such as tea (page 22). For external purposes, a violet-infused tea or lotion (page 28) can be an excellent form of breast care and self-examination.

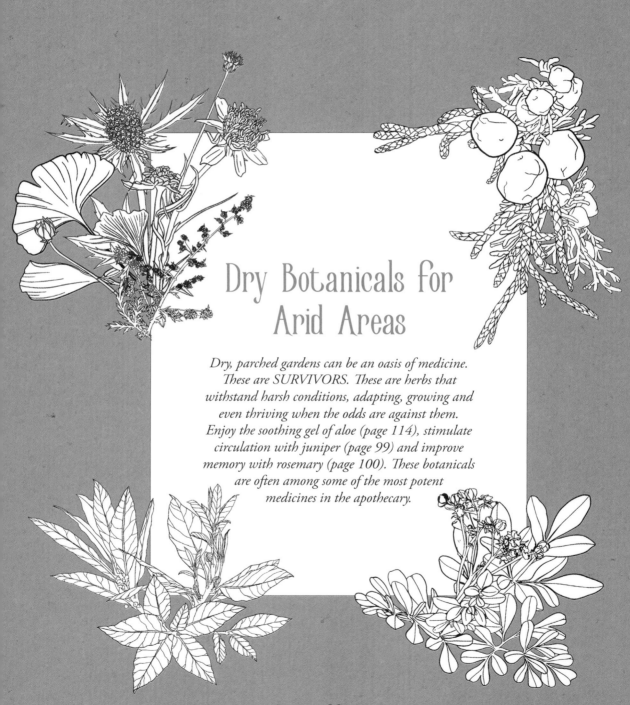

Dry Botanicals for Arid Areas

Dry, parched gardens can be an oasis of medicine. These are SURVIVORS. These are herbs that withstand harsh conditions, adapting, growing and even thriving when the odds are against them. Enjoy the soothing gel of aloe (page 114), stimulate circulation with juniper (page 99) and improve memory with rosemary (page 100). These botanicals are often among some of the most potent medicines in the apothecary.

Agrimony

Agrimonia eupatoria

Herbal Energetics: Cool/dry
Signatures: Steadfast, strong, bold

With its name harkening from the Greek word argemone, *meaning plant to treat the eye, this herb is an excellent remedy for eye complaints such as styes, pink eyes and allergies. Agrimony is considered a remedy for nerve pain, particularly neuropathy of the feet, plantar fasciitis and heel pain. This herb is also greatly cooling and toning to the digestive system and is often used to address GERD symptoms associated with excessive* H. pyroli *in the gut. Agrimony also soothes the mind, calming anxiety for those who find themselves hot, sweaty and even itchy when faced with overwhelm.*

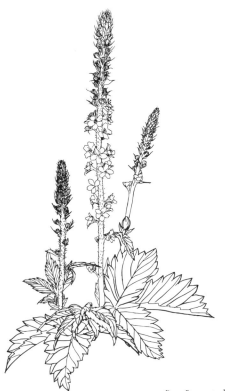

PLANT SNAPSHOT

Perennial
Zone: 6–9
Growth Habit: Mounding with upright flower spikes

GROWING THIS HEALING BOTANICAL

Light Requirements: Full sun

Garden Placement: This herb sends up tall spikes of bright yellow flowers, making it a great choice for the middle to back of a bed or border.

Soil Preference: Agrimony thrives in dry, sandy or rocky soils, as it is prone to root rot and is tolerant of fairly poor fertility.

When to Plant: Sow agrimony seeds directly in prepared soil mid-fall to encourage early spring growth.

Best Growing Tips: Agrimony is a great herb for dry landscapes. Avoid overhead watering when irrigation is needed to prevent powdery mildew.

Garden Companions: Agrimony pairs well with herbs such as rosemary, lavender and thyme.

HARVESTING THIS HERBAL ALLY

Parts Used: Leaves, stem, flowers

When to Harvest for Medicinal Potency: Gather aerial parts of agrimony during the growing season under an ascending moon.

HERBAL REMEDY TIP

Agrimony makes an excellent foot bath when combined with Epsom salts. Place a generous palmful of herbs and a cup of salts into a small container or dedicated foot tub filled with hot water and bathe tender feet until relief comes. For concern of painful and debilitating neuropathy, try an agrimony tincture (page 24).

Yucca

Yucca filamentosa, glauca

Herbal Energetics: Cool/damp
Signatures: Sharp, strong

Yucca is a traditional, if not well known, medicinal herb used to relieve pain and inflammation. This herb may bring comfort to sore, swollen joints and nerve pain. It is considered a blood-purifying, alterative herb and can be used as an ally in illness and addiction recovery. Yucca has a soap-like quality and can be used as a shampoo and body wash, as well as for wound cleansing.

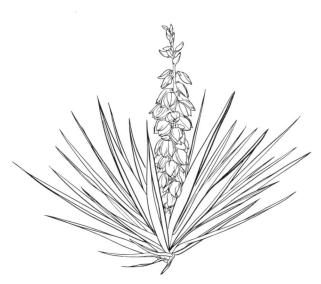

PLANT SNAPSHOT
Shrub or tree
Zone: 5–11
Growth Habit: Straplike mounds, upright flower spike

GROWING THIS HEALING BOTANICAL

Light Requirements: Full sun

Garden Placement: With cultivars growing from 2 feet (0.6 m) to over 30 feet (9 m), choose a spot where yucca has plenty of room to reach its potential.

Soil Preference: Yucca thrives in sandy or gravelly soil with excellent drainage.

When to Plant: Yucca is best propagated by division. Separate volunteers and transplant during a waning moon.

Best Growing Tips: This botanical is an excellent choice for hot spots such as south-facing exposures and against buildings where light and heat reflection is an issue.

Garden Companions: Plant yucca with other succulents like aloe vera and sedums, as well as salvia family herbs.

HARVESTING THIS HERBAL ALLY

Parts Used: Flowers, seed pods (edible), roots (medicinal)

When to Harvest for Medicinal Potency: Dig up roots in early fall during a waning moon.

HERBAL REMEDY TIP

Tincture dried roots (page 24) and use daily to prevent and relieve painful, rheumatic joints.

Juniper

Juniperus communis (avoid *J. savin,* as it is toxic)

Herbal Energetics: Warm/dry
Signatures: Assertive, bold, aggressive

Juniper is a viscerally warming, diffusive herb—this is a fluid mover. Juniper acts specifically on the kidneys and urinary tract system, helping to relieve a congested, boggy bladder and promote kidney health, though it should be avoided during acute infections, as it is powerfully warming. This botanical can reduce limb edema and congested lymph glands, while also rushing blood flow to arthritic joints made stiff by cold and inactivity. Juniper is also a great way to address slow digestion, bloating and gas, making it a great herb to consume prior to a meal.

PLANT SNAPSHOT
Shrub
Zone: 2–7
Growth Habit: Dense, bushy, large

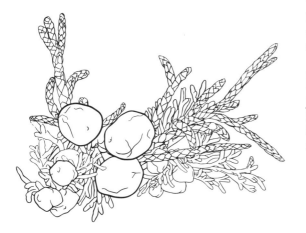

GROWING THIS HEALING BOTANICAL

Light Requirements: Full sun

Garden Placement: Juniper makes a great hedge or barrier in the garden.

Soil Preference: This botanical tolerates dry, sandy, somewhat infertile soil.

When to Plant: Juniper is easily propagated by rooting 4- to 6-inch (10- to 15-cm) branches during a waning moon cycle. Note: Most nursery juniper cultivars are grafted onto specific rootstock to promote certain growth and plant behaviors, so the resulting seedling may develop differently than the parent plant.

Best Growing Tips: Juniper is dioecious, meaning that there are both male and female plants. Select both to produce fertile berries from the female plant. Also note that juniper foliage can be somewhat irritating to the skin, so wear gloves when planting, pruning and harvesting.

Garden Companions: Juniper has allelopathic properties and may discourage some nearby plants, so this botanical is a good choice for planting as a focal point away from others, but may grow peacefully with other evergreens, ornamental grasses and bamboo.

HARVESTING THIS HERBAL ALLY

Parts Used: Berries

When to Harvest for Medicinal Potency: Gather berries during late summer and early fall, when they become dry to the touch, during an ascending moon.

HERBAL REMEDY TIP

Juniper is often used in gin distillation and makes for a great aperitif before dinner. Make a warming, woodsy massage oil by infusing dried berries in an oil of your choice (page 27).

Rosemary

Salvia rosmarinus

Herbal Energetics: Warm/dry
Signatures: Generous, uplifting

In addition to being a favored culinary herb, rosemary is indispensable in the apothecary. Viscerally warming, diffusive and stimulating, this is an herb to light the internal fires. Rosemary increases circulation and raises sluggish blood pressure. It heightens cognitive function and benefits memory, making it a great herb to experience while studying and researching. Rosemary will also stimulate sluggish urination and promote full bladder elimination. It also relieves stressed and exhausted muscles after exertion.

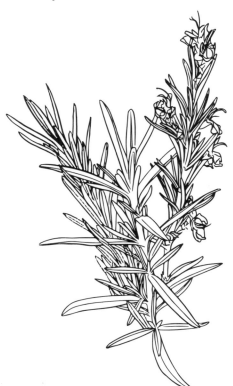

PLANT SNAPSHOT

Evergreen perennial
Zone: 6–10
Growth Habit: Upright or trailing depending on cultivar

GROWING THIS HEALING BOTANICAL

Light Requirements: Full sun

Garden Placement: Rosemary cultivars are gorgeous in rocky gardens and trailing over sunny retention walls.

Soil Preference: Rosemary requires dry, well-draining soils of low to moderate fertility.

When to Plant: Rosemary is most easily propagated by stem cuttings. During a waning moon, remove a 4- to 6-inch (10- to 15-cm) stem, remove two-thirds of the lower leaves and place it in water until roots are well formed. Transplant outdoors after the danger of frost has passed, also during a descending moon.

Best Growing Tips: Rosemary can become woody, so an aggressive harvest of stems around the time of bloom can encourage supple, new growth.

Garden Companions: Rosemary is at home with other Mediterranean herbs like thyme, sage and oregano but will deter pests when planted near brassicas and strawberries.

HARVESTING THIS HERBAL ALLY

Parts Used: Leaves

When to Harvest for Medicinal Potency: Harvest rosemary stems just as they begin to bloom under an ascending moon.

HERBAL REMEDY TIP

Never pass an opportunity to add fresh rosemary to a meal, but for medicinal purposes, a tincture of fresh rosemary (page 24) is ideal for improving clarity and focus when feeling unmotivated and forgetful.

Bay

Laurus nobilis

Herbal Energetics: Warm/dry
Signatures: Sturdy, stately

This botanical is steeped in mythology and ripe with medicinal virtue. Bay is a highly aromatic, pungent herb that is often used for culinary purposes, which is suggestive of its therapeutic actions. Bay settles an upset stomach, invigorates appetite and reduces bloating and flatulence. It has a gentle diuretic action, supporting the kidneys and promoting full bladder elimination. Bay is thought to increase a sense of vitality and wake-fulness, while also providing relief for headaches.

PLANT SNAPSHOT
Shrub
Zone: 8–10
Growth Habit: Woody shrub

GROWING THIS HEALING BOTANICAL

Light Requirements: Full sun to partial shade (provides protection from harsh afternoon rays)

Garden Placement: Bay makes an excellent foundation shrub in an herb garden with its shiny evergreen leaves.

Soil Preference: Bay is tolerant of a variety of soil conditions, as long as the soils are well drained.

When to Plant: Bay is most easily propagated by stem cutting. Cut a 4- to 6-inch (10- to 15-cm) stem, removing all but the topmost leaves. Place the stem in water during a waning moon until the roots have formed. Transplant into soil during a descending moon.

Best Growing Tips: If growing in cooler climates, grow in a container that can be brought indoors during cooler months.

Garden Companions: Plant bay near beans or in the herb garden with rosemary, sage and lavender.

HARVESTING THIS HERBAL ALLY

Parts Used: Leaves

When to Harvest for Medicinal Potency: Gather leaves throughout the summer months during an ascending moon.

HERBAL REMEDY TIP

Infuse bay into bone broth and sip it to aid in illness recovery and increase appetite when feeling feeble, weak and lacking enthusiasm.

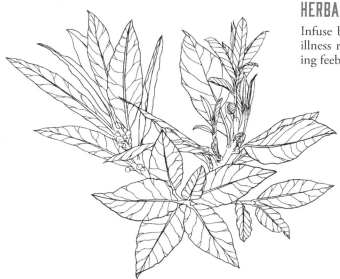

Nigella (Black Seed, Black Cumin)

Nigella sativa

Herbal Energetics: Warm/dry
Signatures: Ethereal, evanescent

Known in the Muslim medicinal tradition as the medicine for everything but death, we can gather the panacea-like effect that nigella (also called "love in a mist") possesses. While it may appear that this botanical is the cure for all that ails, it is particularly useful for those with cold, damp conditions. Nigella has strong antihistamine benefits for allergy sufferers with weeping eyes, persistent sneezing attacks and boggy sinuses. Nigella is particularly useful for digestive complaints, including cramping, diarrhea, bloating, flatulence and colic. There are even emerging studies supporting nigella's anti-cancer and anti-cell proliferate properties, which translates well to home use for boils and cysts.

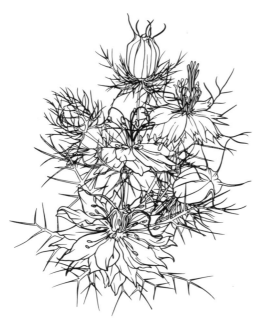

PLANT SNAPSHOT

Free-seeding annual
Zone: 2–10
Growth Habit: Lacy, diminutive

GROWING THIS HEALING BOTANICAL

Light Requirements: Full sun

Garden Placement: This small botanical is exquisite in cottage-type gardens, where it can be placed near the front of borders and beds to be appreciated.

Soil Preference: Nigella prefers light, loamy, well-drained soils of moderate fertility.

When to Plant: Sow nigella seeds 6 to 8 weeks before last frost during a waxing moon. Transplant outdoors after the danger of frost has passed, during a descending moon.

Best Growing Tips: Nigella prefers the cooler edges of the season, so plant for early summer bloom, leaving some seed heads to mature and reseed for a repeat as the weather cools in late summer and early fall.

Garden Companions: Plant nigella with California poppy and calendula where similar growing conditions can be observed.

HARVESTING THIS HERBAL ALLY

Parts Used: Seeds

When to Harvest for Medicinal Potency: Gather seed heads as they mature and brown during an ascending moon.

HERBAL REMEDY TIP

Crush aromatic, nutmeg-scented nigella seeds with honey using a mortar and pestle and create a paste to stir into water for a warming tea (page 22). Sip after a heavy meal to ease digestion.

Wormwood

Artemisia absinthium

Herbal Energetics: Cool/dry
Signatures: Soft, cool, lit from within

Long heralded as a digestive herb, the bitter bite of wormwood stimulates the salivary response to spur digestive action, improving the appetite. This bitter agent aids in the digestion of fats and increases motility in the digestive system. It is considered a tonic for the liver and may be especially useful for those recovering from alcoholic excess. Wormwood also acts as an antiparasitic, ridding the digestive system of worms contracted through tainted water and food.

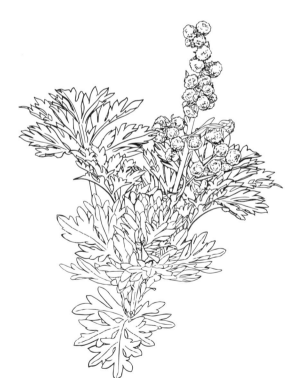

GROWING THIS HEALING BOTANICAL

Light Requirements: Full sun to partial shade

Garden Placement: The soft, light gray-olive tonality of wormwood makes this botanical a remarkable juxtaposition to dark foliage and flowers in beds and container plantings.

Soil Preference: Wormwood needs light, well-draining soils of low to average fertility.

When to Plant: Sow wormwood seeds indoors 6 to 8 weeks before last frost during a waxing moon. Transplant outdoors when danger of frost has passed, during a descending moon.

Best Growing Tips: To maintain a rounded, bushy plant, trim wormwood back to a few inches from the ground in a dome shape in early fall.

Garden Companions: Plant wormwood in the vegetable garden or anywhere that leaf-nibbling insects are a concern.

HARVESTING THIS HERBAL ALLY

Parts Used: Leaves

When to Harvest for Medicinal Potency: Harvest stems of wormwood from plants at least 2 years of age, just as it starts to bloom during an ascending moon.

HERBAL REMEDY TIP

Tincture fresh wormwood (page 24) and take a dose before meals to encourage appetite and suppress bloating and heartburn.

Sea Buckthorn

Hippophae rhamnoides

Herbal Energetics: Warm/dry (leaves) to damp (berries)
Signatures: Resolute, rugged

Sea buckthorn oil is a popular beauty remedy promoting soft, supple and radiant skin. But far from just an herb used for skincare, this botanical offers benefits to the immune, cardiovascular and digestive systems. Sea buckthorn berries are considered a superfood, offering powerful anti-oxidants to prevent viral cell damage, while the whole herb can help reduce a spasmodic cough, asthma symptoms, wheezing and a thick, heaving breath. These antioxidant properties, coupled with its anti-inflammatory benefits, make sea buckthorn a natural support for maintaining healthy cholesterol function, protecting the heart and managing blood pressure. It can also help reduce abdominal cramping, increase appetite for those recovering from illness and support the natural detoxification processes of the body.

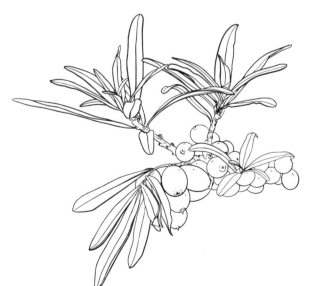

PLANT SNAPSHOT

Shrub
Zone: 2–9
Growth Habit: Large, bushy

GROWING THIS HEALING BOTANICAL

Light Requirements: Full sun

Garden Placement: Sea buckthorn will thrive in conditions where many plants suffer such as near beachside salt spray and cold, shallow, rocky mountainous exposures.

Soil Preference: This botanical is well suited to sandy and rocky conditions and does not require highly nutritive soils, making it a perfect solution for erosion control.

When to Plant: Dig up suckers with healthy roots as they emerge in spring and transplant them during a waning moon. Seeds can be sown in late winter or early spring during an ascending moon, but plants grown from seeds may take up to 4 years to achieve fruiting maturity.

Best Growing Tips: Sea buckthorns are dioecious, meaning that plants are either male or female and a garden will need both to produce fertile berries.

Garden Companions: Sea buckthorn is a suitable companion for wild roses species such as *R. rugosa*, as well as yarrow, rosemary and bay.

HARVESTING THIS HERBAL ALLY

Parts Used: Leaves, berries, seed (as oil extract)

When to Harvest for Medicinal Potency: Gather leaves and berries throughout the fruiting season under an ascending moon.

HERBAL REMEDY TIP

Using fresh, frozen or dried berries and dried leaves, combined with cinnamon and ginger, concoct a tea (page 22) to consume before meals to invigorate a weak appetite or to protect against viral threats.

Thyme

Thymus vulgaris

Herbal Energetics: Warm/dry
Signatures: Comforting, protective

As indispensable in the apothecary as it is in the kitchen, thyme is an herb to open, clear and warm at a deep, visceral level. Thyme is diffusive and antimicrobial in nature, making it a foremost ally to ward off colds, flu and infection. Thyme will clear boggy, congested sinuses and soften hardened mucus—the kind that makes every cough feel like shards of glass are scraping at your throat. Its antispasmodic action relieves both menstrual and digestive cramping, as well as reduces the spasmodic hacking of respiratory complaints such as bronchitis and whooping cough. Thyme can encourage a lackluster appetite and ease digestion.

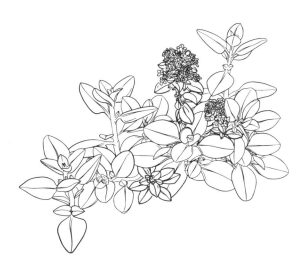

PLANT SNAPSHOT

Perennial
Zone: 2–10
Growth Habit: Low growing ground cover

GROWING THIS HEALING BOTANICAL

Light Requirements: Full sun

Garden Placement: Plant thyme near the front of borders where its diminutive stature will not be overlooked. Some species of thyme make a stepable ground cover between flag stones, pavers and bricks.

Soil Preference: Thyme thrives in light, well-draining soils of poor to average fertility.

When to Plant: The fastest way to propagate thyme is by root division. Simply slicing through the root system of an existing clump, lift a section with sufficient roots and transplant it during a waning moon. Alternatively, thyme seeds can be sown indoors 6 to 8 weeks before last frost during an ascending moon.

Best Growing Tips: When harvesting thyme, cut or beak the stems close to the soil line to encourage thick, lush growth.

Garden Companions: Plant thyme among strawberries to deter pests.

HARVESTING THIS HERBAL ALLY

Parts Used: Leaves, flowers

When to Harvest for Medicinal Potency: Gather thyme under a waxing moon just as it begins to flower.

HERBAL REMEDY TIP

Infuse raw honey (page 26) with copious amounts of thyme to take by the spoonful at the first sign of a sore throat or to sweeten your tea.

Navajo Tea (Hopi Tea/Greenthread/Cota)

Thelesperma subnudum, filifolium (may also be seen as *Cota tinctoria*)

Herbal Energetics: Cool/dry
Signatures: Yielding, open, airy

The varied species of Thelesperma, *commonly called Navajo tea in modern western herbalism, are a highly valued traditional medicine of indigenous Americans. Navajo tea is a digestive aid, improving gallbladder function and assisting in the digestion of fats. This herb also helps expel intestinal parasites. As an antispasmodic, Navajo tea can relieve stomach, intestinal and uterine cramping. Additionally, this botanical contains luteolin and is a wonderful herb for eye health.*

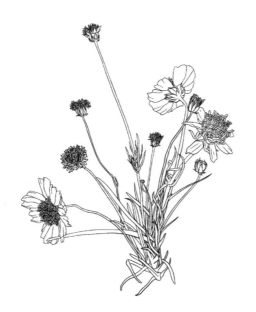

PLANT SNAPSHOT

Short-lived perennial, reseeding annual
Zone: 5–11
Growth Habit: Mounding, tall flower spikes

GROWING THIS HEALING BOTANICAL

Light Requirements: Full sun

Garden Placement: Navajo tea is suited well to xeriscaped gardens and high desert, naturalized landscapes where it can reseed.

Soil Preference: Navajo tea thrives in loose, sandy soils of poor fertility.

When to Plant: Sow seeds directly into prepared soil in fall to allow a natural period of cold stratification.

Best Growing Tips: When sowing directly into a bed, be aware that newly emerged Navajo tea growth is nearly identical to that of grass, so mark your seeded area clearly!

Garden Companions: Navajo tea pairs well with other high-desert dwelling plants like sagebrush.

HARVESTING THIS HERBAL ALLY

Parts Used: Stems, leaves, flowers

When to Harvest for Medicinal Potency: Trim the long flowering stems of Navajo tea as the flowers start to bloom during a waxing moon.

HERBAL REMEDY TIP

Honor the indigenous tradition of bending the long blooming stems of this botanical into bundles that can be snipped as needed and simmered for 5 minutes to extract its aromas and flavors. Slough off some bloom to the simmered decoction to add vibrancy and flavor.

Sea Holly

Eryngium maritimum

Herbal Energetics: Cool/dry
Signatures: Airy, light, wispy

Not widely used in modern herbalism, lovely sea holly was a common apothecary herb in the 17th and 18th centuries. Sea holly was considered an aphrodisiac, perhaps owing this action to its ability to tone reproductive organs and the bladder, thereby reducing a sense of fullness and discomfort about the pelvic region. This herb also supports kidney health and helps with the elimination of stones. Sea holly is thought to stimulate those who feel sluggish and underwhelmed and those prone to procrastination.

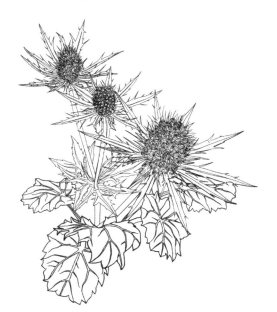

PLANT SNAPSHOT

Perennial
Zone: 4–9
Growth Habit: Arching, tall, somewhat prone to being top heavy

GROWING THIS HEALING BOTANICAL

Light Requirements: Full sun

Garden Placement: Sea holly is a great choice for the middle of a bed or border, boasting grayish foliage and blue flowers, bringing a contrast of color and texture to the landscape.

Soil Preference: Sea holly performs well in sandy soils of poor to moderate fertility and is an excellent choice for coastal areas.

When to Plant: Sow seeds in fall to allow for cold stratification.

Best Growing Tips: Sea holly is ideal in poor soils and can become quite floppy and top heavy in fertile conditions. As such, plant sea holly in areas that receive little care or water.

Garden Companions: Plant sea holly with echinacea, which can provide support for this botanical.

HARVESTING THIS HERBAL ALLY

Parts Used: Roots, leaves, flowers

When to Harvest for Medicinal Potency: Gather roots and flowers as the flowers begin to open during an ascending moon. Dig up roots in the fall under a descending moon.

HERBAL REMEDY TIP

Sea holly is the perfect libido booster for women that often feel a sense of laxity and fullness in the pelvic region that reduces desire. To remedy this, a tincture of sea holly root (page 24) can be taken until libido improves.

Uva Ursi

Arctostaphylos uva-ursi

Herbal Energetics: Cool/dry
Signatures: Protective, generous, stable

Uva ursi is a renowned herb for the renal system. Notably effective for bladder complaints, uva ursi is a remedy for urinary tract infections, enlarged prostate, interstitial cystitis, bladder leakage and urinary retention. This herb may also ease the passage of kidney stones and relieve a sensitivity about the kidneys. It is an effective treatment for excessive vaginal discharge and involuntary erectile complaints. As a diuretic, this herb can greatly diminish a sense of water retention and overall sense of fullness.

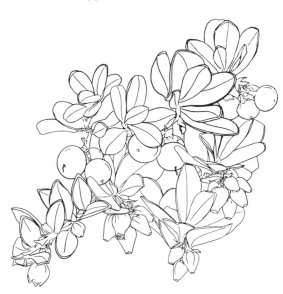

PLANT SNAPSHOT
Shrub
Zone: 2–7
Growth Habit: Woody creeping shrub

GROWING THIS HEALING BOTANICAL

Light Requirements: Full sun

Garden Placement: Uva ursi is a perfect choice for rock gardens, slopes and anywhere soil erosion is a concern.

Soil Preference: This botanical prefers rocky well-drained soils.

When to Plant: Uva ursi is best propagated by cutting a 4- to 6-inch (10- to 15-cm) stem, stripping off the bottom two-thirds of foliage and placing it in water until roots develop. Transplant uva ursi outdoors during a waning moon.

Best Growing Tips: Uva ursi is well adapted to harsh, poor conditions. Do not overwater or overfeed this botanical, as it may result in a week, leggy plant.

Garden Companions: Plant uva ursi with pine, catmint and even sea buckthorn for a rugged medicinal landscape.

HARVESTING THIS HERBAL ALLY

Parts Used: Leaves

When to Harvest for Medicinal Potency: Gather leaves during a waxing moon throughout the growing season.

HERBAL REMEDY TIP

Craft a fresh uva ursi tincture (page 24) and dose at the first sign of bladder discomfort until all irritation has passed.

Ginkgo

Ginkgo biloba

Herbal Energetics: Cool/dry
Signatures: Majestic, unique

This ancient tree has a well-earned reputation for supporting and improving memory. Ginkgo increases cerebral circulation, improving brain health. It decreases cognitive decline and may also uplift those suffering from depression and anxiety. Ginkgo also acts on the respiratory system, decreasing wheezing and relieving asthma complaints, as well as aiding a productive cough to expel mucus from deep in the lungs.

PLANT SNAPSHOT

Tree
Zone: 4–9
Growth Habit: Upright

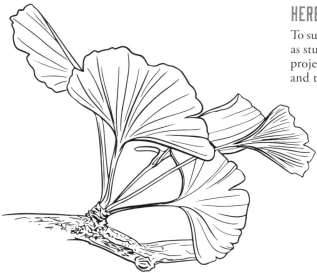

GROWING THIS HEALING BOTANICAL

Light Requirements: Full sun to partial shade

Garden Placement: Plant ginkgo trees where they can reach their full mature size of 50 to 80 feet (15 to 24 m). Ginkgo is tolerant of salt and ocean spray making this a great tree to plant in coastal areas.

Soil Preference: Gingko prefers light loamy or sandy soils of moderate fertility with excellent drainage.

When to Plant: Propagate ginkgo by taking a 4- to 6-inch (10- to 15-cm) cutting. Place it in water until roots form and transplant it during a descending moon.

Best Growing Tips: Ginkgo trees are dioecious. Grow only "male" trees, as female trees produce smelly fruits.

Garden Companions: Ginkgo trees appreciate the same conditions as firs.

HARVESTING THIS HERBAL ALLY

Parts Used: Leaves

When to Harvest for Medicinal Potency: Gather leaves when they are fully open in late spring during an ascending moon.

HERBAL REMEDY TIP

To support clarity and cognition, for activities such as studying for an exam or working on an intense project, create a tincture of ginkgo (page 24) and take it for a period of up to 2 weeks.

Lavender

Lavandula angustifolia, latifolia, x intermedia

Herbal Energetics: Cool/dry
Signatures: Welcoming, cleansing, inviting

Lavender is renowned for the sense of cleanliness and freshness that it evokes, which is substantiated by its antiseptic, antimicrobial and insecticidal benefits. As such, lavender is a perfect herbal choice for cleaning houses, protecting linens and repelling insects. Lavender is profoundly cooling and anti-inflammatory, attributes that are praised in medical fields for burn care. Lavender is a divinely sedative herb, relieving anxiety and promoting restful sleep. This herb also quells a nervous upset stomach, relaxes tension and eases intestinal and uterine cramping.

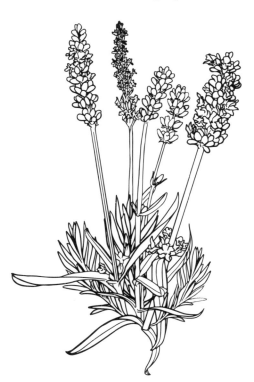

PLANT SNAPSHOT

Perennial
Zone: 5–9
Growth Habit: Mounding, flower spikes

GROWING THIS HEALING BOTANICAL

Light Requirements: Full sun

Garden Placement: Lavender begs to be planted as a long border along footpaths where one can rake their fingers through the blooms and delight in the aromatic bliss.

Soil Preference: Lavender prefers light, well-drained soils of average fertility.

When to Plant: Sow lavender seeds indoors 10 to 12 weeks before the last forest under an ascending moon. Barely cover the seeds and keep them warm. Transplant them outdoors after the danger of frost has passed, during a waxing moon.

Best Growing Tips: To prevent a woody unsightly base, prune lavender wands after its first flush of blooms, and again in early fall, taking it back to a semi-rounded mound.

Garden Companions: Plant lavender with other sun-loving, drought-tolerant herbs such as rosemary, yarrow, sage, oregano and thyme, or near the vegetable garden to lure pollinators!

HARVESTING THIS HERBAL ALLY

Parts Used: Flowers

When to Harvest for Medicinal Potency: Gather flowers as the buds begin to open during an ascending moon.

HERBAL REMEDY TIP

Craft a lavender-infused body oil (page 27) to apply after a shower or bath, before bedtime, to relieve daily strain and gently ease you into a restful slumber.

Rue

Ruta graveolens

Herbal Energetics: Warm/dry
Signatures: Shy, retreating

Rue is a threshold herb, one that invites but does not exclaim. As such, it teaches us to use it as a gateway herb. This bracingly bitter herb is a profound insect repellent that can deter flies, ants and other invaders from the home. Rue breaks up and moves chronic stagnation and can be used where there are concerns of chronic amenorrhea, delayed menses and sluggish digestion. Rue remains one of the more esoteric herbs, considered a low-dose botanical, balancing the masculine and feminine. Herbalists outside of a magical tradition tend to look to this herb for normalizing hormonal imbalance.

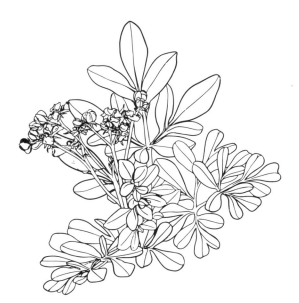

PLANT SNAPSHOT

Perennial
Zone: 4–9
Growth Habit: Upright, mounding

GROWING THIS HEALING BOTANICAL

Light Requirements: Full sun

Garden Placement: Plant rue in pots on a sunny threshold to deter insects and prevent ill will from entering the home.

Soil Preference: Rue requires loose soils of adequate drainage of poor to moderate fertility.

When to Plant: Sow rue seeds indoors 6 to 8 weeks before last frost, during a waxing moon. Transplant the seedlings outdoors when the average daily temperature is approximately 70° F (21°C) during a descending moon.

Best Growing Tips: Propagate rue mid- to late summer by trimming 4- to 6-inch (10- to 15-cm) stems and removing lower stems. Place naked stems in water until roots are well developed. Transplant outdoors when danger of frost has passed during a waning moon.

Garden Companions: As an insect deterrent, plant rue near any susceptible vegetation.

HARVESTING THIS HERBAL ALLY

Parts Used: Leaves, flowers

When to Harvest for Medicinal Potency: Harvest the blooming tips of rue under an ascending moon just as the plants start to bloom.

HERBAL REMEDY TIP

I plant rue in a pair of pots outside of any household threshold, especially where pets might linger and rest to decrease pests.

Oregano

Origanum vulgare

Herbal Energetics: Warm/dry
Signatures: Generous, prolific

Oregano is relegated to the herbs and spices cabinet of many kitchens but offers more than flavor! An intensely warming herb, oregano is also diffusive in action, helping to break up stagnant conditions. As such, oregano is ideal for stodgy, damp sinuses and congestion, as well as nausea caused by sinus drainage into the stomach. Oregano is an excellent herb for slow digestion and those with bacterial concerns in the digestive system. This herb will invigorate blood flow and help to loosen stiff, achy joints.

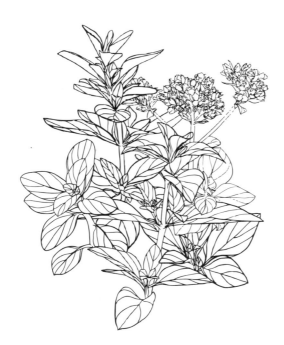

PLANT SNAPSHOT

Perennial
Zone: 5–10
Growth Habit: Upright or somewhat creeping, medium height groundcover

GROWING THIS HEALING BOTANICAL

Light Requirements: Full sun

Garden Placement: Oregano is best placed where it has room to spread. Depending on the cultivar, it may be very low growing or up to 18 inches (46 cm) in height. It can serve as a fragrant ground cover.

Soil Preference: This botanical prefers drier soils of poor to moderate fertility.

When to Plant: Sow oregano seeds indoors 6 to 8 weeks before last frost during an ascending moon, or existing clumps can be easily divided in spring and transplanted during a waning moon.

Best Growing Tips: Oregano can quickly take over an area, so harvest frequently throughout the growing season.

Garden Companions: Plant oregano near tomatoes to deter pests or with other dry-loving botanicals like lavender, rosemary and thyme.

HARVESTING THIS HERBAL ALLY

Parts Used: Leaves, flowers

When to Harvest for Medicinal Potency: Harvest the lush foliage just as it starts to bloom during an ascending moon.

HERBAL REMEDY TIP

For those healing from gastric distress such as food poisoning, a virus or an ulcer, infuse a hearty bone broth with a generous amount of oregano and sip daily or use as a base of soups to heal the gut and promote digestion.

Sweet Alyssum

Lobularia maritima

Herbal Energetics: Cool/dry
Signatures: Generous, sweet, kind

The sweet, honey-scented blooms of sweet alyssum offer a host of benefits. This herb is cooling and astringent, making it a great common cold remedy when there are complaints of sinus drainage with a sense of heat in the throat. It is a mild diuretic, relieving a congested bladder and sense of fullness about the kidneys. Sweet alyssum is also thought to soften those prone to fits of anger and rage.

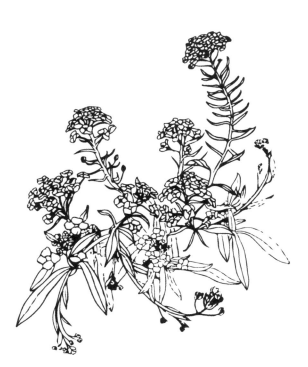

PLANT SNAPSHOT

Annual
Zone: 1–12
Growth Habit: Mat-like, low growing

GROWING THIS HEALING BOTANICAL

Light Requirements: Full sun to light shade (where afternoon sun is especially aggressive)

Garden Placement: Sweet alyssum produces a mat-like ground cover and is perfect for underplanting taller botanicals and is best positioned towards the front of a bed or border.

Soil Preference: Sweet alyssum prefers moderately fertile, well-draining, somewhat dry soils.

When to Plant: Sow sweet alyssum seeds indoors 4 to 6 weeks before last frost during a waxing moon. Transplant seedlings outdoors after all danger of frost has passed, during a descending moon.

Best Growing Tips: Shear sweet alyssum after the first flowering to encourage another flush of growth and bloom in late summer.

Garden Companions: Plant sweet alyssum near botanicals that are susceptible to aphids, such as roses, where it will attract predatory insects.

HARVESTING THIS HERBAL ALLY

Parts Used: Leaves, flowers

When to Harvest for Medicinal Potency: Harvest leaves and flowers during an ascending moon just as the flowers begin to open.

HERBAL REMEDY TIP

In times of frustration and anger such as career trouble and relationship turmoil, create a flower essence by placing your cut sweet alyssum in distilled water for 2 to 3 days. Preserve the strained infusion with a tablespoon (15 ml) of 100-proof spirits. Take three to five drops of this essence when you feel the heat of anger rising and invite sweetness into your life.

Aloe

Aloe vera

Herbal Energetics: Cool/moist
Signatures: Fleshy, full

The cooling gel of aloe is renowned for soothing red, inflamed conditions. Aloe is particularly effective as a remedy for sunburn, providing almost immediate relief from irritation and pain. It is also a great additive into facial care when the surface of the skin is dehydrated, ashy and prone to flaking and can be used to address dandruff and hair loss. Aloe will also soften scabs and help prevent the formation of scars. Internally, aloe can cool heat in the digestive system such as heartburn and relieve constipation.

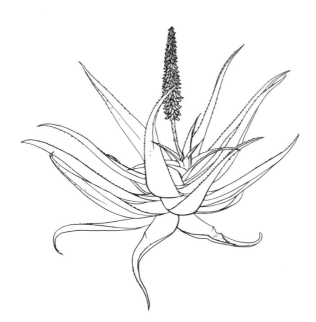

PLANT SNAPSHOT

Succulent shrub
Zone: 8–11 (can be grown as a houseplant in cooler regions)
Growth Habit: Upright, spikey

GROWING THIS HEALING BOTANICAL

Light Requirements: Full sun

Garden Placement: Aloe is a great choice for xeriscaped and rock gardens in warm growing zones.

Soil Preference: Aloe requires dry, sandy or gravelly soils and excellent drainage.

When to Plant: Aloe is best propagated by "pups," small secondary plants growing off the mother plant. Remove the pups and allow the bases to dry and callous (if roots are not present) for a couple of weeks before then planting them in succulent potting mix deep enough to support the plant structure during a descending moon.

Best Growing Tips: Aloe makes a wonderful houseplant placed quite near a sunny window for those living outside aloe's native desert growing region.

Garden Companions: Aloe grows very well with alliums like garlic, onions and shallots.

HARVESTING THIS HERBAL ALLY

Parts Used: Gel expressed from the inside of cut leaves

When to Harvest for Medicinal Potency: Trim leaves as needed during an ascending moon.

HERBAL REMEDY TIP

Aloe leaves can be trimmed and the gel expressed, which can then be frozen in ice cube trays for future use. This makes an excellent remedy to minor burns sustained in the kitchen!

Black Walnut

Juglans nigra

Herbal Energetics: Cool/dry
Signatures: Strong, dominant

The towering black walnut tree provides powerful medicine packed in the outer husk of its nuts. Black walnut is profoundly antifungal and is one of the most effective remedies against ringworm and other fungal complaints of the sick. It may also clear acne and breakout-prone, oily skin. It is also used when there are concerns of intestinal parasites. Additionally, black walnut is a rare source of botanical, land-based iodine and can be useful in addressing mild iodine deficiency hypothyroidism.

PLANT SNAPSHOT

Tree
Zone: 4–9
Growth Habit: Upright, tall

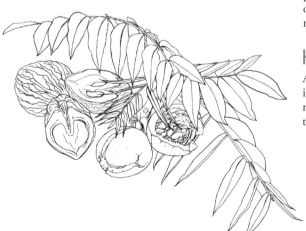

GROWING THIS HEALING BOTANICAL

Light Requirements: Full sun

Garden Placement: Black walnuts have allelopathic properties due to high juglone, meaning that they greatly discourage other vegetation within their vicinity. As such, they are best planted alone where they have room to reach their mature height and reach.

Soil Preference: Black walnuts are adaptive to a variety or soil conditions, but thrive in relatively dry, gritty, sandy soils of modest fertility.

When to Plant: Plant black walnut seeds (the nut in its shell) in the fall under approximately 2 inches (5 cm) of soil.

Best Growing Tips: When growing black walnuts for nut production, prune the upward growth to promote branching.

Garden Companions: While this botanical discourages many botanicals from growing nearby, elderberry, witch hazel and sweet woodruff are all juglone resistant.

HARVESTING THIS HERBAL ALLY

Parts Used: Hulls (outer fleshy coating), nuts (edible)

When to Harvest for Medicinal Potency: Gather fallen nuts in late summer and early fall, particularly during a new moon. Slough off the outer greenish hull, wearing gloves to salve for medicine making.

HERBAL REMEDY TIP

A salve (page 27) created from black walnut–infused oil (page 27), is the single most effective remedy for ringworms that I have ever encountered!

Pine

Pinus species

Herbal Energetics: Slightly warm/slightly dry
Signatures: Adaptive, strong, capable, protective

Pine is reputable as an immune system stimulant, warming and encouraging our body's natural defenses. Its diaphoretic action can help break a low grade, persistent fever. Pine also acts as a mild diuretic, relieving complaints of full bladders and sore kidneys. Pine can relieve the pain associated with exertion, cold exposure and illness. Bathing in pine can reduce general body odor and the persistent scent of stink that one may experience after illness or addiction detoxification/recovery. Pine resin is considered "nature's bandage," protecting wounds from exposure, while also drawing slivers, splinters and lodged debris.

PLANT SNAPSHOT

Tree
Zone: 3–9
Growth Habit: Upright, tall

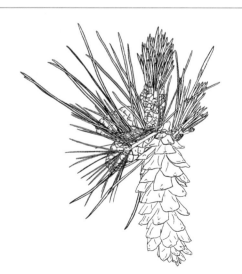

GROWING THIS HEALING BOTANICAL

Light Requirements: Full sun

Garden Placement: Give pines room to grow to their full potential free from neighboring trees, structures and powerlines. Pines are adaptive to the harsh conditions of desert, mountainous and seaside regions.

Soil Preference: Pines prefer dry soils of low to moderate fertility.

When to Plant: Gather fallen cones in the fall and allow them to dry. Tap to dislodge seeds from the bracts of the cone and place them in a bowl of water; only floating seeds are viable. Sow seeds indoors in early spring during an ascending moon.

Best Growing Tips: To grow a straight-trunked tree, pines need a lot of sun exposure. If a certain exposure is too shaded, young pines will lean toward the direction of greater sun.

Garden Companions: Pine grows well in similar conditions as junipers, sea buckthorn and yarrow.

HARVESTING THIS HERBAL ALLY

Parts Used: Needles, pollen, inner bark, resin, nuts (edible)

When to Harvest for Medicinal Potency: Harvest fresh growing tips when they are bright green in early spring during an ascending moon. Cut resin from outer bark when slightly hard to touch (leaving a layer to protect the "wound" in the tree). Inner bark can be scraped from fallen branches. Collect fallen cones in autumn for pine nuts.

HERBAL REMEDY TIP

A sachet of pine needles added to a bath brings a relaxing, aromatic soak to leave your body feeling limber, calm and delightfully perfumed, which is perfect after recovering from the stagnancy of illness and being bedridden.

Yarrow

Achillea millefolium

Herbal Energetics: Neutral/balancing
Signatures: Persistent, rewarding, generous

Yarrow is undoubtedly one of the most useful herbs in the apothecary. Yarrow has a unique ability to staunch the flow of blood from relatively minor cuts, while its antimicrobial action cleans and disinfects the wound. Yarrow is a truly balancing herb, helping the body to achieve a stasis and healthy neutrality. This herb is often employed from concerns of the female reproductive system, both encouraging delayed menses while also reducing excessive menstrual flow. Yarrow can soothe excessive heat in the digestive system while promoting strong digestive action. This herb will also stimulate perspiration to reduce a hot, sudden fever, while also breaking one that is sluggish with associated clamminess.

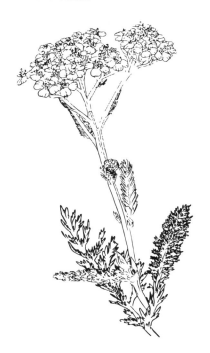

PLANT SNAPSHOT

Perennial
Zone: 3–9
Growth Habit: Ferny, open

GROWING THIS HEALING BOTANICAL

Light Requirements: Full sun

Garden Placement: Yarrow's delicate foliage and array of colors, from white to the deepest burgundy blooms, make it a gorgeous addition to the midsection of cottage and Mediterranean borders.

Soil Preference: Yarrow prefers light, well-drained, even sandy beachside soils.

When to Plant: Sow yarrow seeds indoors 6 to 8 weeks before last frost during an ascending moon. Transplant outdoors after the danger of frost has passed during a descending moon.

Best Growing Tips: In its favored conditions, yarrow can become slightly invasive and crawl into lawns. Harvest freely during bloom to avoid the spread.

Garden Companions: Yarrow is thought to increase the aromatics of neighboring plants while also deterring pests from tender plants such as roses and garden vegetables.

HARVESTING THIS HERBAL ALLY

Parts Used: Flowers

When to Harvest for Medicinal Potency: Gather flowers as they are fully open during an ascending moon.

HERBAL REMEDY TIP

Infuse yarrow in witch hazel extract (follow the cold infusion method on page 23), strain and pour into a spray bottle for emergency herbal first aid. Spray liberally in and around the wound site and experience the fast-healing potential of this wonderful herb.

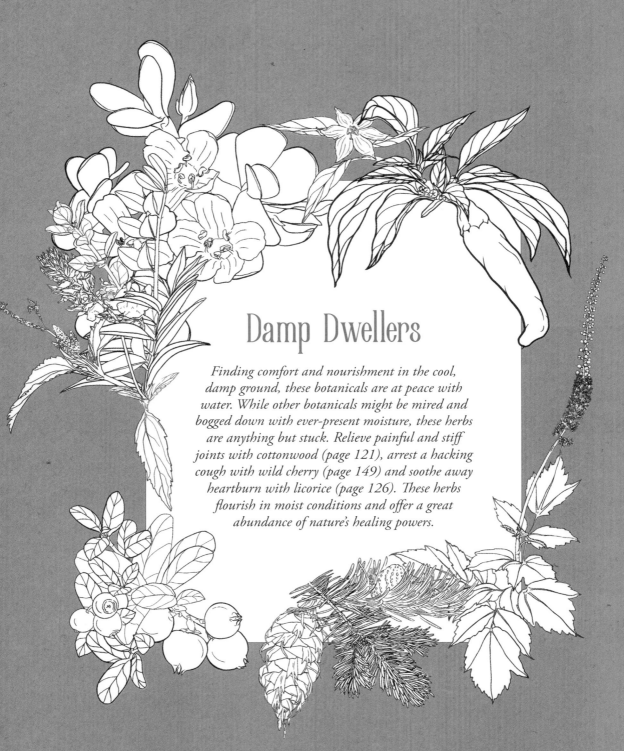

Damp Dwellers

Finding comfort and nourishment in the cool, damp ground, these botanicals are at peace with water. While other botanicals might be mired and bogged down with ever-present moisture, these herbs are anything but stuck. Relieve painful and stiff joints with cottonwood (page 121), arrest a hacking cough with wild cherry (page 149) and soothe away heartburn with licorice (page 126). These herbs flourish in moist conditions and offer a great abundance of nature's healing powers.

Birch

Betula alba, benta, papyrifera, platyphylla var japonica, pendula

Herbal Energetics: Cool/dry
Signatures: Dramatic, guiding

Birch is a forest ally offering a host of medicinal properties. This botanical is an excellent pain reliever, owing to its methyl salicylate constituent, making it effectively one of nature's aspirins (like cottonwood and willows). Highly astringent, birch can prove helpful with eruptive and oozy skin conditions like acne, eczema and weepy sunburns. Additionally, birch supports healthy blood sugar and relieves inflammation.

PLANT SNAPSHOT

Tree
Zone: 3–8
Growth Habit: Tall, straight (although some species may be multi-trunked and more shrub-like)

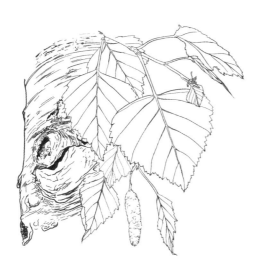

GROWING THIS HEALING BOTANICAL

Light requirements: Full sun to partial shade

Garden Placement: Plant birches where they can achieve their species or cultivar size potential. The striking white, peeling bark helps to radiate light and energy in a woodland garden with other darker foliaged botanicals.

Soil Preference: Birches like moderately rich, deep, silty moist soil.

When to Plant: Birches are most easily propagated from stem cuttings. Remove all the foliage except for the topmost leaves. Place the stem in water until roots form. Plant outdoors under a waning moon.

Best Growing Tips: Especially during establishment, birches have a new and ample supply of water, so they are ideal for growing near river and creek sides, and even boggy or swampy soils.

Garden Companions: Birches are fast growing and ideal for sheltering fragile botanicals that are prone to sunburn.

HARVESTING THIS HERBAL ALLY

Parts Used: Bark, twigs, leaves

When to Harvest for Medicinal Potency: Gather leaves when they are fully open in the spring under an ascending moon. Gather twigs and bark from fallen limbs, ideally dropped in spring storms when the tree is at its most medicinal.

HERBAL REMEDY TIP

Birch emits the most wonderful wintergreen aroma from spring-harvested foliage and bark. Brew a decoction of birch bark (page 23) and let it cool. Then, soak a towel or cloth with the decoction to apply around angry, hot joints irritated by exertion and stress.

Cornflower

Centaurea cyanus

Herbal Energetics: Cool/dry
Signatures: Crownlike, jeweled

Cornflower has been used historically for concerns of the eye. As an astringent herb, cornflower soothes red, itchy, inflamed eyes, styes, blepharitis, conjunctivitis and even dark circles and black eyes. It acts as a mild diuretic and can help with a sense of kidney fullness and urinary retention, as well as support digestion and liver function. Additionally, cornflower is an excellent remedy for oily and dandruff-prone scalps.

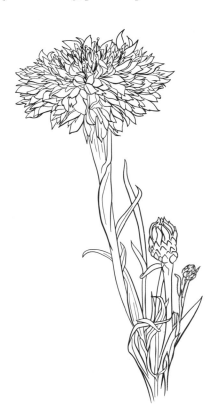

PLANT SNAPSHOT

Perennial
Zone: 4–8
Growth Habit: Sprawling, open

GROWING THIS HEALING BOTANICAL

Light Requirements: Full sun to partial shade

Garden Placement: Cornflowers spread freely and are well suited to a lush cottage garden.

Soil Preference: This botanical performs well in average, well-drained soils but needs frequent watering to promote lush foliage and bloom.

When to Plant: Sow seeds indoors 6 to 8 weeks before the last frost during an ascending moon. Transplant outdoors after the danger of frost has passed, under a waning moon. Divide existing clumps and transplant them in the fall during a descending moon.

Best Growing Tips: Cornflowers can become scrawny and leggy looking if not deadheaded/harvested and trimmed and should be divided every 2 to 3 years.

Garden Companions: Plant with bee balm for a bright display or pollinator-friendly flowers.

HARVESTING THIS HERBAL ALLY

Parts Used: Leaves, flowers

When to Harvest for Medicinal Potency: Gather leaves and flowers as the blooms open throughout the growing season during an ascending moon.

HERBAL REMEDY TIP

Create a poultice of fresh cornflower blooms to apply to puffy, swollen eyes. Rest fully reclined for 15 to 20 minutes before rinsing eyes with cool water and enjoying a revitalized visage.

Cottonwood

Populus trichocarpa

Herbal Energetics: Cool/dry
Signatures: Towering, resilient

The sweet, honey-like aroma of late winter cottonwood bud resin is like the clarion call for herbalists to start wildcrafting after winter's rest. Cottonwood has been long considered one of nature's "cure-alls" because it offers so much in the way of pain relief, wound healing and immune-supporting benefits. Containing the same constituents that are the active ingredient of aspirin, cottonwood is a great pain reliever. It is also a stimulating expectorant capable of bringing up deep lung junk. Cottonwood promotes wound healing by reducing instances of inflammation.

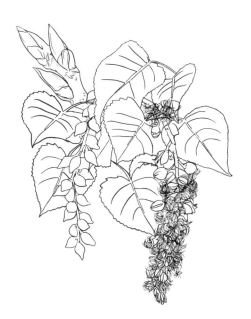

PLANT SNAPSHOT
Tree
Zone: 2–9
Growth Habit: Tall, upright

GROWING THIS HEALING BOTANICAL

Light Requirements: Full sun to partial shade

Garden Placement: Cottonwoods are best planted near waterways and near natural springs where water is abundant.

Soil Preference: Cottonwoods are ideally suited to wet, boggy soils that are moderately rich.

When to Plant: Cottonwoods are most easily propagated by cuttings. Cut a 4- to 6-inch (10- to 15-cm) stem leaving the two topmost leaves and place it in water until roots develop. Transplant the cutting under a waning moon.

Best Growing Tips: Cottonwoods are the perfect choice for areas that are perpetually wet and problematic for other botanicals.

Garden Companions: Underplant cottonwood with stinging nettle for a perfect woodland medicinal expanse.

HARVESTING THIS HERBAL ALLY

Parts Used: Bark, buds

When to Harvest for Medicinal Potency: Gather fallen buds and bark from windfall as they present themselves.

HERBAL REMEDY TIP

Dry cottonwood buds thoroughly and infuse them in oil (page 27) with cayenne for a deeply penetrating joint pain relief salve. Apply liberally and often to provide an increased sense of flexibility and movement.

Cayenne

Capsicum annuum

Herbal Energetics: Warm/dry

Signatures: Bold, aggressive, non-apologetic

This intensely hot herb is perfectly suited for bringing cold conditions to a comfortable neutral. Cayenne is an excellent pain reliever for achy arthritic joints, particularly those irritated by cold and damp weather. As a rubefacient, cayenne will bring color and warmth to the surface of the skin. Internally, this herb invigorates the appetite and encourages fluid consumption. Cayenne is highly stimulating and can loosen an unproductive heavy cough, relieve a sense of bloating and fullness, soothe sore muscles and ease menstrual cramps.

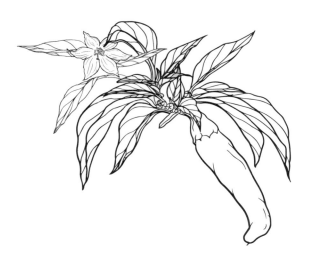

PLANT SNAPSHOT

Perennial

Zone: 9–11 (grown as an annual elsewhere)

Growth Habit: Bushy

GROWING THIS HEALING BOTANICAL

Light Requirements: Full sun

Garden Placement: Plant cayenne in a warm spot in the garden where access to irrigation can be had.

Soil Preference: Cayenne needs well-drained but moisture-retentive soils of moderate to rich fertility.

When to Plant: Sow cayenne seeds indoors 8 to 10 weeks before the last frost under a waxing moon. Transplant outdoors after the danger of frost has passed during a descending moon.

Best Growing Tips: Cayenne needs both heat and water to thrive. As such, make plans for irrigation to maintain a balance of these conditions.

Garden Companions: Plant cayenne near basil, dill or nasturtiums to deter pests.

HARVESTING THIS HERBAL ALLY

Parts Used: Fruits (peppers), seeds

When to Harvest for Medicinal Potency: Gather cayenne peppers as they redden, especially during a waxing moon.

HERBAL REMEDY TIP

Infuse oil (page 27) with dried cayenne to use as a base for a salve (page 27) to warm cold, stiff, painful joints.

Corydalis

Corydalis aurea, ambigua, canadensis, yanhusuo

Herbal Energetics: Warm/dry
Signatures: Delicate, tender

Corydalis is considered a blood mover in traditional Chinese medicine. As such, it is a botanical that invigorates cold, damp conditions of the body such as slow or arrested digestion, uterine fullness with dysmenorrhea, cramping, water retention and lover stagnation. Known as a very effective pain reliever, corydalis is particularly effective against migraines that are associated with fluctuating hormones. It is also a profoundly effective sedative, promoting a swift retreat into slumber.

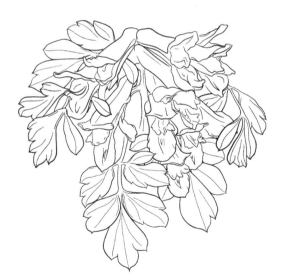

PLANT SNAPSHOT
Perennial
Zone: 5–7
Growth Habit: Mounding

GROWING THIS HEALING BOTANICAL

Light Requirements: Partial to full shade

Garden Placement: Place corydalis in shady woodland gardens close to footpaths and seating areas where delicate foliage and flowers can be enjoyed.

Soil Preference: Corydalis thrives in moderately rich, loamy, moisture-retentive soil. This soil should drain well and not be boggy or swamp-like.

When to Plant: Sow seeds directly into prepared soil mid-fall or divide clumps in early spring and transplant them during a descending moon.

Best Growing Tips: Deadhead spent flowers and cut back leggy foliage to promote new growth and prolific rebloom throughout the growing season.

Garden Companions: As many species of corydalis like to bloom in spring and early summer and start to die back somewhat thereafter, plant with botanicals like hostas and cohosh that come on more boldly later in the season.

HARVESTING THIS HERBAL ALLY

Parts Used: Tuberous rhizome

When to Harvest for Medicinal Potency: Lift and divide corydalis in early fall as the foliage has begun to recede. Harvest the rhizomes under a waning moon.

HERBAL REMEDY TIP

Tincture corydalis root (page 24) and combine with tinctures of California poppy (page 51) to create a slightly sedating remedy for those who suffer from nerve pain and restlessness.

Hawthorn

Crataegus species

Herbal Energetics: Cool/dry
Signatures: Protective, generous

A medicine of the heart, hawthorn heals and protects the cardiovascular system. Hawthorn normalizes blood pressure, both reducing high blood pressure and elevating low blood pressure. This herb supports excellent circulation, reduces blood cholesterol and helps maintain a steady strong heartbeat. On a spiritual and emotional level, hawthorn helps during times of grief and sadness and is ideally suited for the very real sensation of a broken heart.

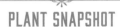

PLANT SNAPSHOT

Tree
Zone: 5–9
Growth Habit: Bushy, shrub-like tree

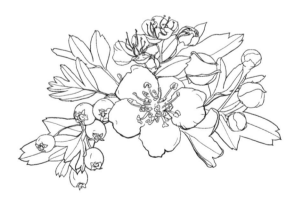

GROWING THIS HEALING BOTANICAL

Light Requirements: Full sun to light shade

Garden Placement: Hawthorn is best placed near the back of beds and borders or wide open spaces. Hawthorn is also ideally suited as a security hedge due to the painful thorns.

Soil Preference: Hawthorns thrive in slightly acidic, moderately fertile, moisture-retentive soils.

When to Plant: Hawthorn seeds need about 365 days to germinate but are often successful when patience is observed. Sow seeds in the spring or fall during an ascending moon and mark the area clearly.

Best Growing Tips: During establishment, stake hawthorn to promote an erect trunk.

Garden Companions: Plant hawthorns and cramp bark together for a showy grouping of medicinal herbs that offer visual excitement throughout the year.

HARVESTING THIS HERBAL ALLY

Parts Used: Leaves, flowers, berries, thorns (esoteric uses)

When to Harvest for Medicinal Potency: Gather leaves and flowers in early spring and berries and thorns in the fall, during an ascending moon.

HERBAL REMEDY TIP

Consider hawthorn a heart healer and boundary setter. Sip a tea (page 22) of hawthorn leaves and flowers steeped with a singular thorn while committing to care and love for yourself, while setting healthy boundaries with others to prevent stress and heartache.

Wild Ginger

Asarum canadense

Herbal Energetics: Warm/dry
Signatures: Secretive, unassuming

Wild ginger is spicy and stimulating, making it ideal for cold, sluggish, damp conditions. Wild ginger viscerally warms the body and increases perspiration, making it a remedy for low fevers when the person feels cold, clammy and prone to shivering chills. It may also help to open clogged, stodgy sinuses. Wild ginger will soothe an upset stomach by draining the sinuses and targeting sluggish digestion. This herb is also stimulating to the female reproductive system, bringing on a slow or delayed menses and clearing a sense of fullness and cramping in the pelvis.

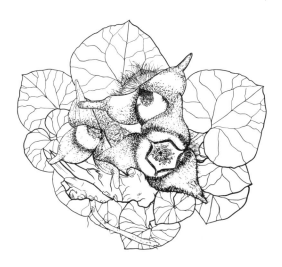

PLANT SNAPSHOT

Perennial
Zone: 3–8
Growth Habit: Diminutive, clumping

GROWING THIS HEALING BOTANICAL

Light Requirements: Full to partial shade

Garden Placement: Plant wild ginger in cool shady areas near the front of a bed or border where this small botanical can be appreciated.

Soil Preference: Wild ginger prefers humus-rich, damp soils.

When to Plant: Divide existing clumps of wild ginger in spring to transplant during a descending moon.

Best Growing Tips: Wild ginger likes damp conditions and can be attractive to slugs and snails. Clear leaf litter and mulch away from the base of the plant and sprinkle diatomaceous earth to prevent damage to foliage.

Garden Companions: Wild ginger grows well in the dense shade of fir and maple trees.

HARVESTING THIS HERBAL ALLY

Parts Used: Rhizome (leaf is toxic)

When to Harvest for Medicinal Potency: Dig and harvest the fleshy rhizomes in late summer during a waning moon.

HERBAL REMEDY TIP

With some concerns of aristolochic acid toxicity when combined with alcohol, the best way to use wild ginger is to use the dried root in a warming tea (page 22) to stimulate sluggish digestion and relieve painful cramping.

Licorice

Glycyrrhiza glabra

Herbal Energetics: Cool/moist
Signatures: Lacy, soft

Licorice is one of the greatest soothers available in the modern herbal pharmacopeia. Licorice helps to restore damaged mucous membranes by coating them with a cooling mucilage. It is a premier treatment for ulcers in the digestive system and is a top treatment for a sore throat with a hot barking cough, such as experienced with strep throat. Licorice is also considered to be among the family of adaptogen herbs and can be used to nourish the adrenal system.

PLANT SNAPSHOT

Perennial
Zone: 7–10
Growth Habit: Clumping

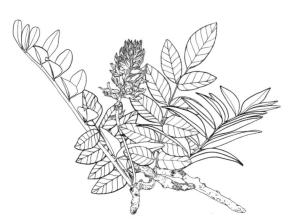

GROWING THIS HEALING BOTANICAL

Light Requirements: Full sun to partial shade

Garden Placement: Licorice is slow to establish, but 2- to 3-year-old plants may grow up to 3 feet (0.9 m) tall and wide, so plant near the back of a bed or border with ample space to reach its potential.

Soil Preference: This botanical prefers slightly alkaline soils that are moisture-retentive but have adequate drainage.

When to Plant: Sow seeds indoors 6 to 8 weeks before the last frost during an ascending moon and keep warm (approximately 68°F [20°C]). Transplant outdoors when all danger of frost has passed under a waning moon.

Best Growing Tips: Licorice is a bit temperamental, needing adequate moisture but is prone to rot, rust and mildew if kept damp. As such, amend denser soil with sand or vermiculite and avoid overhead watering.

Garden Companions: Plant licorice with rosemary, lettuces and calendula.

HARVESTING THIS HERBAL ALLY

Parts Used: Rhizome

When to Harvest for Medicinal Potency: Dig and harvest long rhizomes in early to mid-fall under a descending moon.

HERBAL REMEDY TIP

Licorice is an extremely sweet herb that is a perfect, adjunct herb in adaptogenic and anti-inflammatory formulas. Tincture (page 24) licorice root with turmeric to remedy ulcerative conditions of the digestive system.

Marshmallow

Althaea officinalis

Herbal Energetics: Cool/moist
Signatures: Gentle, soft, welcoming

Marshmallow is perhaps one of the most comforting remedies in the apothecary for hot, dry, cracked and brittle conditions. This herb soothes and protects the mucous membranes of the respiratory and digestive systems. Marshmallow can relieve a sore, raw throat with a painful, sharp cough, while also being an outstanding treatment for ulcerations of the esophagus, stomach and intestines. Externally, marshmallow can soften dry, dehydrated skin prone to flakiness and ashiness.

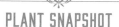

PLANT SNAPSHOT

Perennial
Zone: 3–9
Growth Habit: Mounding, clumping

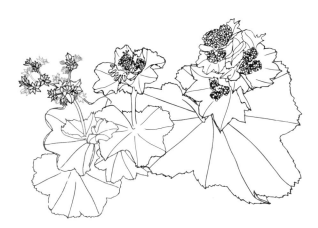

GROWING THIS HEALING BOTANICAL

Light Requirements: Full sun to partial shade

Garden Placement: Marshmallow can grow relatively large and should not be crowded by competing plants. Place marshmallow near the back of a bed or border or in a dedicated bed.

Soil Preference: This botanical is well adapted to moderately fertile, heavy, clay-like soils that retain ample moisture but are not swamp-like.

When to Plant: Direct sow marshmallow seeds in late winter or early spring when at least 6 weeks of cold weather are in the forecast.

Best Growing Tips: Harvesting the roots of this botanical may be easier if it is planted in a raised bed.

Garden Companions: Violets thrive in the cool, moist conditions created by the larger marshmallow plant.

HARVESTING THIS HERBAL ALLY

Parts Used: Roots

When to Harvest for Medicinal Potency: Dig up roots in early fall during a descending moon just as the plant starts to die back.

HERBAL REMEDY TIP

Infuse the marshmallow root in cool water (page 23) to maximize its emollient and demulcent properties. Use this infusion as the aqueous addition to lotions and cream or drink an ounce (30 ml) day and night to soothe and protect acidic stomach complaints.

Mugwort

Artemisia vulgaris

Herbal Energetics: Warm/dry
Signatures: Unassuming, gentle, open

Mugwort is a bitter herb with a sage-like aroma that is well regarded by herbalists for its benefits to the digestive system. This botanical promotes the secretion of gastric juices that increase digestive function, while also increasing bowel regularity and decreasing gas and bloating. It is also a remedy for menstrual complaints such as pelvic fullness, cramping with sharpness, shooting back and anal pain. Mugwort is also a relaxing nervine herb that eases tension and may increase vivid and even lucid dreaming.

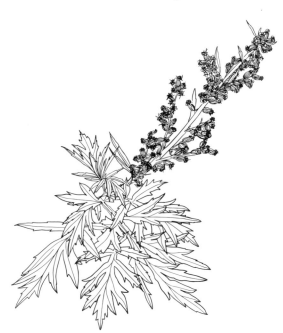

PLANT SNAPSHOT
Perennial
Zone: 4–8
Growth Habit: Sprawling

GROWING THIS HEALING BOTANICAL

Light Requirements: Full sun to partial shade

Garden Placement: Mugwort's open foliage and impressive height of up to 6 feet (1.8 m) suggest that it is best placed toward the back of a bed or border.

Soil Preference: Mugwort is adaptive to a variety of poor conditions, including dry and poor fertility, but thrives in moderate, rich, moisture-retentive soils. This botanical becomes more drought tolerant when well established.

When to Plant: Mugwort is best propagated by root division. Dig and separate existing clumps in early spring as the foliage emerges and transplant divisions during a descending moon.

Best Growing Tips: Mugwort responds well to aggressive harvests throughout the growing season. The aromatics of this herb can be increased by allowing the soil to dry between watering once the plant is well established.

Garden Companions: Due to its full size and deer-repellent nature, plant mugwort around botanicals susceptible to wildlife grazing.

HARVESTING THIS HERBAL ALLY

Parts Used: Leaves

When to Harvest for Medicinal Potency: Harvest the top third of the mugwort throughout the growing season during an ascending moon.

HERBAL REMEDY TIP

Tincture fresh mugwort (page 24). Take the tincture before a meal to increase digestion or before bed to maximize dreaming potential. Keep a journal bedside to record your mugwort-induced dreams!

Elder

Sambucus caerulea, canadenis, nigra

Herbal Energetics: Cool/dry (flower), damp (berries)

Signatures: Abundance, inviting

Elderflowers and elderberries are one of the most useful herbs in the healing apothecary. Elderflowers act as a relaxing diaphoretic, gently cooling heightened fevers while also acting as a potent antiviral to help fight infection. Elderflowers also cool a sense of heartburn associated with acid reflux. Elderberries have long been considered one of the most effective preventative herbs for the cold and flu season. Elderberries also improve digestive function and are a mild laxative.

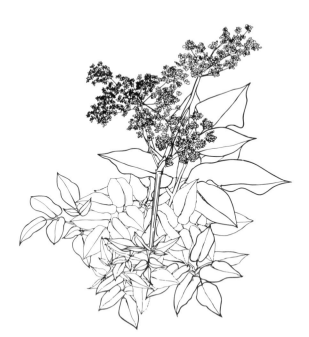

PLANT SNAPSHOT
Tree/shrub
Zone: 3–9
Growth Habit: Multi-trunked tree, growing to tree stature

GROWING THIS HEALING BOTANICAL

Light Requirements: Partial shade to full sun

Garden Placement: Plant elders where they can reach the species and cultivar size potential.

Soil Preference: Elders like moderately rich, loamy or silty moisture-retentive soils.

When to Plant: Elders are most easily propagated by cutting. Cut a 4- to 6-inch (10- to 15-cm) stem, preserving the leaf nodes and place in water until roots form.

Best Growing Tips: When you have a nigra species or "black" elders, plant at least two different cultivars to promote pollination.

Garden Companions: Elders are at home in a watery woodland setting with nettle and cottonwoods.

HARVESTING THIS HERBAL ALLY

Parts Used: Flowers, berries

When to Harvest for Medicinal Potency: Gather flowers in early summer during an ascending moon. Harvest berries in early fall during a waning moon.

HERBAL REMEDY TIP

Sip elderflower tea (page 22) at the first sign of cold or flu until symptoms subside. A syrup of elderberries (page 25) can be taken daily through the cold and flu season and anytime one feels that their immune system may be at risk.

Goldenseal

Hydrastis canadensis

Herbal Energetics: Cool/dry
Signatures: Offering, uplifting

Goldenseal is greatly regarded in the herbal apothecary as an herb for infections, particularly those that are bacterial in nature. This botanical is ideal for sinus infections—both clearing the infection and normalizing the flow of mucus. In the digestive system, goldenseal is thought to be effective against H. pylori *(a common comorbidity with peptic ulcers). It is also thought to be effective against certain sexually transmitted infections, excessive vaginal discharge, diarrhea and dysentery.*

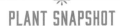

PLANT SNAPSHOT

Perennial
Zone: 3–8
Growth Habit: Upturned, palmlike

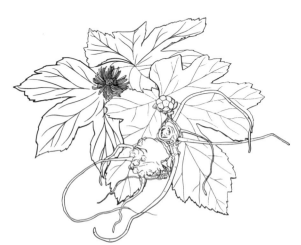

GROWING THIS HEALING BOTANICAL

Light Requirements: Partial shade

Garden Placement: Grow goldenseal in shady landscapes towards the front of the border or bed.

Soil Preference: This botanical prefers moderately rich, loamy, moisture-retentive soils.

When to Plant: Seed propagation is difficult and inconsistent at best, so it is best to propagate goldenseal via root division. In late fall, dig up an existing clump and trim the rhizomes with feeder rootlets. Snip them into 1-inch (2.5-cm) sections with feeder rootlets and transplant them during a descending moon.

Best Growing Tips: Native wild goldenseal has been devastated by over-harvesting, so growing your own supply is the only ethical way to use this herb.

Garden Companions: Plant goldenseal with ginseng, black cohosh and beth root.

HARVESTING THIS HERBAL ALLY

Parts Used: Roots, leaves, flowers, fruits

When to Harvest for Medicinal Potency: Gather aboveground parts during the summer months, during an ascending moon. Dig and harvest the rhizomes in early fall under a waning moon.

HERBAL REMEDY TIP

In years past, it was more conventional to use only the root, but modern herbalists suggest using the whole plant in tincture form (page 24). Harvest the various parts of goldenseal at the height of potency and combine the finished tinctures after infusion is complete.

Cranberry

Vaccinium macrocarpon

Herbal Energetics: Cool/dry
Signatures: Abundant

As an antiseptic diuretic, cranberries are perhaps foremost known for their ability to treat urinary tract infections, while also supporting healthy renal function. Cranberries are high in antioxidants, which neutralize free radicals, thereby protecting cells from microbial invaders and cellular damage. This same antioxidant action also supports the cardiovascular system and promotes healthy blood cholesterol levels.

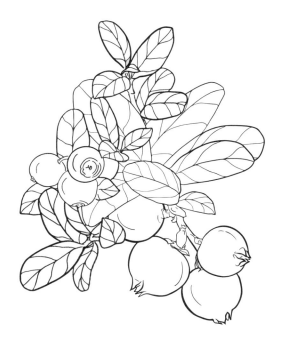

PLANT SNAPSHOT

Perennial
Zone: 2–8
Growth Habit: Upright, shrub-like

GROWING THIS HEALING BOTANICAL

Light Requirements: Full sun

Garden Placement: Unlike images of cranberry bogs (flooded to facilitate commercial harvest), cranberries grow well in fertile, moisture-retentive garden soil.

Soil Preference: Cranberries thrive in highly acidic, fertile, silty moisture-retentive soils.

When to Plant: Cranberries are most easily propagated by cuttings; trim a 6- to 8-inch (16- to 20-cm) cutting from a plant that is at least 3 years old. Remove all but the top four leaves and sink the stem in water until roots are established. Transplant cuttings outside under a waning moon.

Best Growing Tips: Cranberries have high nutritional needs and supplemental nitrogen may help to produce upright shoots.

Garden Companions: Grow cranberries near other acid-loving plants such as blueberries.

HARVESTING THIS HERBAL ALLY

Parts Used: Berries

When to Harvest for Medicinal Potency: Gather berries in the fall as the berries redden during an ascending moon.

HERBAL REMEDY TIP

While unsweetened cranberry juice is often used to address urinary complaints, a tincture of fresh cranberries (page 24) will confer similar benefits.

Gravel Root (Joe Pye Weed)

Eutrochium purpureum

Herbal Energetics: Cool/dry
Signatures: Rising, elevating

Gravel root is great for the kidneys and is one of the best treatments in the apothecary for kidney stones. This botanical seems to not only assist in the passing of kidney stones, but may also prevent the formation of them in the first place, making it an excellent herb for those with recurring kidney complaints. It also relieves kidney edema and pain while promoting full bladder elimination. Gravel root may also benefit those suffering from rheumatism and gout, as well as menstrual complaints of cramping and endometriosis.

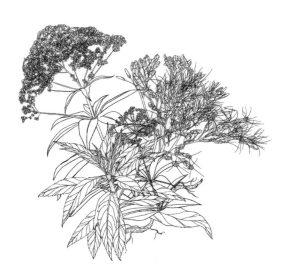

PLANT SNAPSHOT

Perennial
Zone: 4–8
Growth Habit: Tall, erect

GROWING THIS HEALING BOTANICAL

Light Requirements: Full sun to partial shade

Garden Placement: Plant gravel root near ponds and streams or in damp areas of the landscape, taking into account the towering 5- to 7-feet (1.5- to 2.1-m) stature of this botanical.

Soil Preference: Gravel root prefers moderately rich soils that remain consistently moist, but not swamp-like.

When to Plant: Gravel root is best propagated by root division. Dig up and divide clumps in spring as new foliage starts to emerge and transplant during a waning moon.

Best Growing Tips: Prune dying and spent foliage in early fall as the plant starts to die back so that the next year's foliage is clear of dead and decaying material.

Garden Companions: Gravel root grows well near elecampane and vervain.

HARVESTING THIS HERBAL ALLY

Parts Used: Root

When to Harvest for Medicinal Potency: Dig up roots in early fall as the plant starts to die back during a descending moon.

HERBAL REMEDY TIP

Tincture fresh gravel root (page 24) and take when the first sign of tenderness about the kidneys presents itself; continue taking daily until all signs of tenderness pass.

Lovage

Levisticum officinale

Herbal Energetics: Warm/dry
Signatures: Lush, inviting

Lovage's flavor can best be described as spicy celery, which is suggestive of its therapeutic actions in the body. Lovage is used for "irrigation therapy" to help flush the body of toxins. The warm, spicy flavor and salinity of lovage encourages thirst, while its strong diuretic action promotes urination. This two-fold effect benefits those with chronic kidney and bladder complaints, edema, water retention, gout and rheumatism. Additionally, lovage lights the digestive "fire" and increases the peristaltic action of the stomach. It also promotes delayed menses and relieves menstrual cramping with a sense of bogginess about the pelvic region.

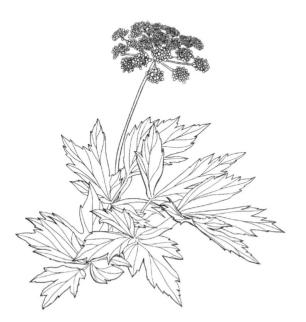

PLANT SNAPSHOT

Perennial
Zone: 3–9
Growth Habit: Bushy with tall flower spikes

GROWING THIS HEALING BOTANICAL

Light Requirements: Full sun to partial shade

Garden Placement: Lovage can grow quite lush and tall and should be planted toward the midsection or the back of a bed, border or container.

Soil Preference: Lovage thrives in rich, loamy, moisture-retentive soils.

When to Plant: Sow lovage seeds indoors 4 to 6 weeks before the last frost during an ascending moon.

Best Growing Tips: Lovage thrives in relatively cool conditions and the soil should be kept consistently moist to prevent leaf bitterness.

Garden Companions: Plant lovage amongst root crops such as potatoes and beets.

HARVESTING THIS HERBAL ALLY

Parts Used: Leaves, stems

When to Harvest for Medicinal Potency: Gather leaves and tender stems throughout the summer during a waxing moon.

HERBAL REMEDY TIP

Incorporate lovage into your fresh herb repertoire for meals or create an infusion (page 22) to use as the liquid addition to green smoothies with spinach and avocado, especially if you find yourself with a cold constitution with sluggish digestion. Accompany lovage use with LOTS of fresh water to maximize its benefits.

Bacopa

Bacopa monnieri

Herbal Energetics: Cool/damp
Signatures: Gentle, unassuming

Bacopa is often overlooked as a medicinal in the garden. Far from a simple botanical, bacopa is a powerful ally for brain health and neurological function. This herb contributes to a heightened sense of well-being, ability to adapt to stressors and increases one's ability to feel joy. Bacopa is thought to improve cognitive function, specifically increase short-term memory retention. As such, the herb is ideal for students, those with hectic work and home and those with age-related memory-retention complaints.

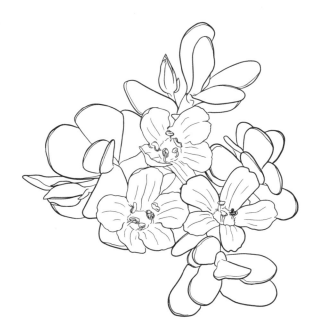

PLANT SNAPSHOT

Perennial
Zone: 8–11
Growth Habit: Creeping, trailing

GROWING THIS HEALING BOTANICAL

Light Requirements: Full sun to partial shade

Garden Placement: This creeping botanical is ideal for hanging baskets or containers, but also makes an excellent ground cover.

Soil Preference: Bacopa likes moderately rich, slightly acidic, moisture-retentive soils.

When to Plant: Bacopa is most easily propagated by stem cuttings. Trim a 4- to 6-inch (10- to 15-cm) stem and remove the bottom two-thirds of the leaves. Place it in water during a waning moon until the roots form. Transplant to prepared soil when roots are well developed.

Best Growing Tips: Brown leaves are a sign of iron deficiency in bacopa. Lowering the pH of the soil while supplementing may help with nutrient uptake.

Garden Companions: Bacopa is an ideal botanical for container gardens and baskets and does well with the likes of lamb's ear and lady's mantle.

HARVESTING THIS HERBAL ALLY

Parts Used: Leaves, stems and flowers

When to Harvest for Medicinal Potency: Gather the flowering tips and leaves of bacopa during an ascending moon.

HERBAL REMEDY TIP

Tincture bacopa (page 24) and take it daily to increase a sense of well-being and adaptability in the fast-paced modern world.

Linden

Tilia americana

Herbal Energetics: Cool/moist
Signatures: Sheltering, supple, soft

Linden is a beautifully uplifting herb—one that is ideal for those who feel stressed and brittle, cracking around the edge. It helps greatly to dial down surging cortisol levels to moderate the body's physiological response to stress. It is gently sedative in action, without making one feel drowsy, making it ideal for those who feel like they can't shake their workload at the end of the day. Linden is excellent for addressing rapid heartbeat and palpitations. It also supports the immune system and can soothe a hot, dry, inflamed throat and a sharp, painful cough.

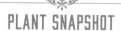

PLANT SNAPSHOT

Tree
Zone: 3–8
Growth Habit: Upright, pyramidal to oval-shaped canopy.

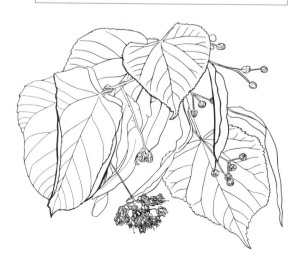

GROWING THIS HEALING BOTANICAL

Light Requirements: Full sun to light shade

Garden Placement: Lindens are slowly growing trees that may eventually reach a height of 35 to 50 feet (10.5 to 15 m) but are slow to achieve that size. Keep its potential in mind when planting and avoid potential obstacles in its path or growth.

Soil Preference: Linden is highly adaptable to a variety of soil conditions but requires moisture-retentive soils with good drainage to help avoid withering and browning.

When to Plant: Seed propagation of linden is tricky and unreliable, so it is best to dig up a volunteer sapling and transplant it under a waning moon.

Best Growing Tips: Lindens are noncompetitive trees, meaning that they won't thrive when densely planted with more aggressive botanicals. Plant this tree where it has room to establish such as more open areas.

Garden Companions: Linden is a great attractor of pollinators, so plant this tree near the vegetable garden to promote a bountiful harvest.

HARVESTING THIS HERBAL ALLY

Parts Used: Leaves, flowers

When to Harvest for Medicinal Potency: Gather leaves and flowers as they begin to open during an ascending moon. Prone to ants, give your harvest a good shake and leave it outside for a few hours where the insects can scurry away before bringing it inside to dry.

HERBAL REMEDY TIP

Do your heart and mind a favor. Create a tea of linden and hawthorn (page 22) to enjoy after a stressful day—this makes an excellent remedy instead of turning to alcohol to unwind.

Mimosa

Albizia julibrissin

Herbal Energetics: Cool/dry
Signatures: Ethereal, tender, otherworldly

While many herbs address depression, stress and anxiety, it is mimosa that is heralded for times of intense grief and heartache. Mimosa helps to balance adrenal hormones that become off kilter during times of great emotional despair. Its antioxidant action protects the heart and nourishes the cardiovascular system. Additionally, this botanical is gently sedative and can send the mind and body into a relaxing slumber when the mind is overwrought with sadness.

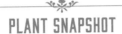

PLANT SNAPSHOT

Tree
Zone: 6–9
Growth Habit: Upright, somewhat shrubby if not pruned during early establishment.

GROWING THIS HEALING BOTANICAL

Light Requirements: Full sun

Garden Placement: Plant mimosa trees where they can spread and reach their potential without obstruction and where it won't be overly shaded by larger trees. Note that this tree is invasive in some regions.

Soil Preference: Mimosa is somewhat opportunistic and can thrive in poor, clay-like disturbed soils and near roadsides if the soil is moisture retentive.

When to Plant: This tree grows easily from seed. Sow seeds indoors in sunny, warm locations after scuffing the seeds with a file or rasp and soaking them overnight during an ascending moon.

Best Growing Tips: Mimosas are somewhat prone to limb breakage due to heavy winds and ice, so it is ideal to plant them where there is some break from significant gusts. While quite breathtaking in bloom, it drops a significant volume of spent flowers and leaf litter, so keep that in mind if one prefers a "tidy" landscape.

Garden Companions: Mimosa fixes nitrogen in the soil and can provide increased nutrition for heavy feeding botanicals such as corn, basil, coriander and parsley.

HARVESTING THIS HERBAL ALLY

Parts Used: Flower

When to Harvest for Medicinal Potency: Gather flowers in full bloom during a waxing moon.

HERBAL REMEDY TIP

Tincture fresh mimosa blossoms (page 24) to have on hand when times of sorrow and grief occur. Mimosa will help your mind and body understand that it can withstand the pain of loss.

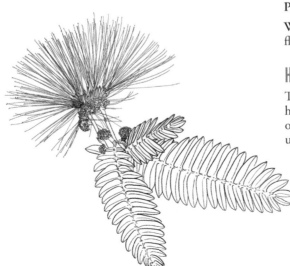

Skullcap (American)

Scutellaria lateriflora

Herbal Energetics: Cool/dry
Signatures: Protective

The helmet-like form of skullcap flowers is suggestive of its action—this is a remedy of a busy and overburdened mind. Skullcap helps to relieve panic attacks and anxiety, particularly for those who feel hot, flustered and overstimulated with a rapid pulse. It is ideal for those in moments of shock and can help one stay calm and make sense of distressing situations. Skullcap also soothes tight, spasmed muscles and it's great for acute persistent pain such as a toothache or minor, irritating injury when there is a constant sense of discomfort and overwhelm.

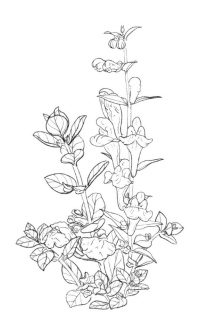

PLANT SNAPSHOT
Perennial
Zone: 4–8
Growth Habit: Upright, mounding

GROWING THIS HEALING BOTANICAL

Light Requirements: Full sun

Garden Placement: Place skullcap toward the midsection or back of the border where it will not be shaded by larger botanicals but can receive ample water.

Soil Preference: Skullcap needs moisture-retentive soils of moderate fertility to thrive.

When to Plant: Sow skullcap seeds indoor for 6 to 8 weeks before last frost during a waxing moon. Transplant outdoors after all danger of frost has passed during a descending moon.

Best Growing Tips: As a member of the mint family, skullcap has a tendency to spread and is ideal for naturalizing into a damp, open meadow landscape that receives plenty of sunlight.

Garden Companions: Flowering throughout the entire growing season, skullcap is a great attractor of pollinators and predatory insects, so plant skullcap around the vegetable garden.

HARVESTING THIS HERBAL ALLY

Parts Used: Leaves, stems, flowers

When to Harvest for Medicinal Potency: Harvest the top third of skullcap throughout the long flowering season as the plant blooms during an ascending moon.

HERBAL REMEDY TIP

If you are plagued with persistent panic attacks or are just a general type A personality, tincture fresh skullcap (page 24) and keep it with you at all times to dial down the overstimulated response.

Valerian

Valeriana officinalis

Herbal Energetics: Warm/dry
Signatures: Gentle, cloudlike

Valerian has long been considered a premier for sleep and restfulness. This herb induces a sleepy, almost hypnotic state and is excellent for those of cold constitution that find themselves persistently unable to fall asleep but does not result in a groggy stupor upon waking. It is ideal for those who have stiff and spasmodic muscles, especially with cold extremities. Valerian is also useful for menstrual cramps and a cold, wet, phlegmy cough.

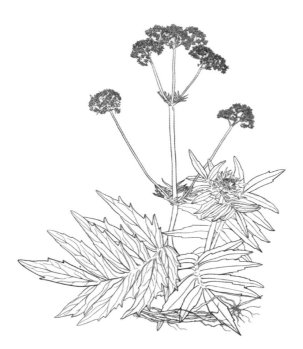

PLANT SNAPSHOT
Perennial
Zone: 4–9
Growth Habit: Clumping, tall

GROWING THIS HEALING BOTANICAL

Light Requirements: Full sun to partial shade

Garden Placement: Valerian can grow quite big and tall and self-seeds with reckless abandon so give it space to expand or place it in a damp area that you want to fill in.

Soil Preference: Valerian likes moderately fertile, silty or loamy, evenly moist but not boggy soils.

When to Plant: Valerian can grow quickly from seed planted directly in the garden after all danger of frost has passed during an ascending moon.

Best Growing Tips: This botanical is carefree and can withstand full sun, but if given afternoon shade, it will absolutely flourish.

Garden Companions: Grow valerian with mints to produce a full and lush medicinal border that will attract pollinators.

HARVESTING THIS HERBAL ALLY

Parts Used: Roots

When to Harvest for Medicinal Potency: Dig up roots after the first frost of fall during a descending moon.

HERBAL REMEDY TIP

The roots of dried valerian have an aroma not unlike damp gym socks, so it is ideally taken quickly as a tincture (page 24). As a tea, it might be unpleasant to sip.

Vervain

Verbena hastata, officinalis

Herbal Energetics: Cool/dry
Signatures: Uplifting, focused, reaching

Vervain is a botanical for the chronically stressed and overburdened mind. It is a particularly effective herbal remedy for those who tend to hyper-focus on tasks, become strictly schedule oriented and overly control situations. It eases those who may find it difficult to change course or perspective into a more holistic frame of mind. It is particularly good for those suffering from muscle stiffness, especially for neck-ache and those who are plagued with tension headaches and insomnia. It also helps strengthen oral and digestive tissues that are inflamed and prone to bleeding.

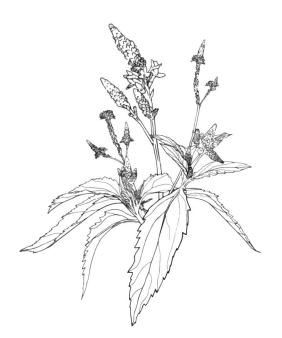

PLANT SNAPSHOT

Perennial
Zone: 3–9
Growth Habit: Erect

GROWING THIS HEALING BOTANICAL

Light Requirements: Full sun to partial shade

Garden Placement: Plant vervain next to ponds and waterways where it can thrive in cool moist soils.

Soil Preference: Vervain prefers a rich silt that is moisture retentive.

When to Plant: Sow seeds directly into prepared soils in early fall.

Best Growing Tips: Vervain responds well to the frequent harvest of the flowering tops throughout the growing season, offering repeat blooms until late summer.

Garden Companions: Vervain grows beautifully side by side with marshmallow.

HARVESTING THIS HERBAL ALLY

Parts Used: Leaves, flowers

When to Harvest for Medicinal Potency: Harvest leaves and flowering tops of vervain as the blooms start to open throughout the growing season during an ascending moon.

HERBAL REMEDY TIP

Tincture fresh vervain (page 24) and use it as a long-term tool to aid in the ability to "let things go" and become more adaptive to the inevitable changes and obstacles that seem to derail life.

Stinging Nettle

Urtica dioica

Herbal Energetics: Cool/dry
Signatures: Abundance, fierce

Quite possibly one of the most useful herbs in herbal pharmacopeia, stinging nettle revitalizes and sharpens the mind, body and spirit. Nettle is packed with vitamins and minerals that restore imbalance and improve overall wellness. This botanical is a remedy for internal "spring cleaning," acting as a diuretic to flush the kidneys and bladder, while promoting bowel elimination if eaten. Nettle can be used to address chronic urinary tract complaints and benign prostatic hyperplasia. Nettle can also be taken preceding and during the allergy season to lessen the severity of hay fever.

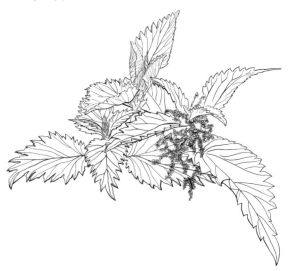

PLANT SNAPSHOT
Perennial
Zone: 4–10
Growth Habit: Upright

GROWING THIS HEALING BOTANICAL

Light Requirements: Partial to full shade

Garden Placement: Stinging nettle is irritating to the touch, so plant it in a dedicated bed to avoid unintended contact.

Soil Preference: Nettle prefers moderately rich, moist soils and can thrive in silty areas near waterways.

When to Plant: Sow nettle seeds directly in prepared soils 3 to 4 weeks before last frost under an ascending moon.

Best Growing Tips: Because the stinging silica barbs covering the stem and the undersides of leaves are incredibly irritating to the touch, wear gloves and long sleeves whenever caring for or harvesting a nettle patch.

Garden Companions: Nettle is thought to increase the essential oil content of nearby plants and makes a suitable companion for aromatic herbs.

HARVESTING THIS HERBAL ALLY

Parts Used: Leaves, seeds

When to Harvest for Medicinal Potency: Using gloved hands (or by pinching the top side of the leaf and pulling), harvest the tops of nettle in early spring during an ascending moon. Gather seeds in summer when they become dry to the touch, during a waxing moon.

HERBAL REMEDY TIP

Allergy sufferers can reduce the severity of their symptoms by taking a tincture of nettle (page 24) as a prophylactic remedy before and during the worst part of their allergies. Blanched nettle makes a flavorful and nutritious alternative to spinach in baked dishes, soups and stews.

Black Cohosh

Actaea racemosa

Herbal Energetics: Cool/dry
Signatures: Graceful, ethereal

Black cohosh has long been favored for women's health concerns from the onset of menstruation through and after menopause. Black cohosh is useful for helping to regulate cycles, reduce heavy flow, lessen breast tenderness and relieve cramping. Later in life, this botanical helps to address fibrous breast tissue, vaginal atrophy and dryness, hot flashes and depression. It may also improve milk flow in nursing mothers. Additionally, black cohosh is a strong antispasmodic, relieving muscle cramps, sciatica, stomach and intestinal griping, and irritable cough.

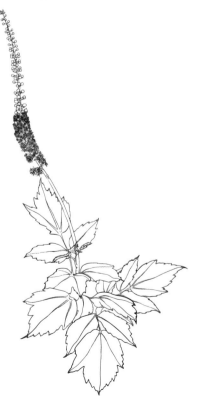

PLANT SNAPSHOT

Perennial
Zone: 4–8
Growth Habit: Tall, arching flower spires

GROWING THIS HEALING BOTANICAL

Light Requirements: Partial to full shade

Garden Placement: Black cohosh is a beautiful addition to a woodland or shade garden producing tall, fragrant white flower spikes.

Soil Preference: Black cohosh prefers deep, humus-rich soils that are moisture-retentive.

When to Plant: This botanical is most easily propagated by rhizome division. Dig and separate the rhizome mass in early spring or mid-fall and transplant the division during a waning moon.

Best Growing Tips: Black cohosh is prone to sun scorching during drought-like conditions, so take special care to plant where this botanical can be protected from the harsh afternoon sun and where its roots can remain cool and moist.

Garden Companions: Black cohosh plays well with other water-loving botanicals like blue flag iris, elderberry and violet.

HARVESTING THIS HERBAL ALLY

Parts Used: Rhizomes

When to Harvest for Medicinal Potency: Dig up and divide rhizomes in early to mid-fall during a descending moon.

HERBAL REMEDY TIP

Tincture fresh black cohosh root (page 24). Consider the far-reaching, long-term benefits of this herb and how it is a tool in the commitment to self-care.

Crampbark

Viburnum opulus

Herbal Energetics: Cool/dry
Signatures: Bright, cheery

As its common name suggests, crampbark is an herb to relieve cramping—everything from muscle exertion pain, to uterine cramping, to irritable cough, to heart palpitations, this is a profoundly antispasmodic herb. Crampbark does this all by stimulating movement of stagnation in fluids in the body. Crampbark is often used by midwives and expectant mothers to reduce uterine irritation and help discern between false (or prodromal labor) and actual active labor. Beyond its anti-spasmodic qualities, crampbark also supports healthy blood pressure and is particularly helpful for type A, nervous types.

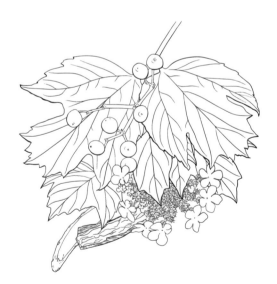

PLANT SNAPSHOT

Tree/shrub
Zone: 3–8
Growth Habit: Bushy, low-growing tree or massive shrub

GROWING THIS HEALING BOTANICAL

Light Requirements: Partial shade to light sun

Garden Placement: Crampbark is a foundation shrub that makes a bold statement in a sheltered bed or border.

Soil Preference: Crampbark prefers moderately rich, moisture-retentive soils.

When to Plant: Because crampbark seeds can take up to 18 months to germinate, crampbark is most easily propagated by cuttings. Trim a 4- to 6-inch (10- to 15-cm) stem, trimming away all but the topmost leaves and place it in water. When roots are well established, transplant it outdoors during a waning moon.

Best Growing Tips: Crampbark should be planted in a somewhat sheltered area where it has ample water and is protected from drying winds.

Garden Companions: Underplant crampbark with low growing, water-loving ground covers like violet and bugleweed.

HARVESTING THIS HERBAL ALLY

Parts Used: Bark

When to Harvest for Medicinal Potency: Peel bark from broken and pruned limbs preferably during an ascending moon.

HERBAL REMEDY TIP

Tincture crampbark (page 24) and take 2 days before the onset of menstrual cramp systems until the day of the cycle, after which symptoms usually pass.

Lady's Mantle

Alchemilla mollis, vulgaris

Herbal Energetics: Cool/dry

Signatures: Curving, resilient, cloaking, protective

Lady's mantle is an herb of balance and restoration. Long held as a "woman's herb," this botanical is thought to help regulate one's cycle and manage menstrual flow, as well as reduce irritation and heat in delicate tissues. While it is well-known for its feminine benefits, lady's mantle offers much more. This herb encourages cellular health, making it a wonderful ingredient in skin preparations to soothe burning, itching, wounds and even cystic acne, while also enhancing skin elasticity and firmness. Additionally, this elegant botanical promotes digestive and respiratory health by helping reduce excessive phlegm and maintain healthy blood pressure, while also supporting good renal and urinary health.

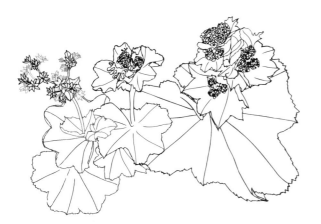

> ## PLANT SNAPSHOT
> Perennial
> **Zone:** 3–8
> **Growth Habit:** Low growing, mounding

GROWING THIS HEALING BOTANICAL

Light Requirements: Light shade or full sun if water supply is adequate

Garden Placement: Plant near the front of borders and along paths where its subtle beauty can be enjoyed.

Soil Preference: Lady's mantle prefers slightly moist loamy soil with a neutral pH and modest fertility

When to Plant: Sow seeds during a waxing moon phase and plant seedlings during a waning moon phase.

Best Growing Tips: Lady's mantle requires adequate moisture for vigor and performance but is otherwise quite a carefree plant. Plant lady's mantle densely to encourage cool, moist conditions that promote healthy root growth.

Garden Companions: Plant with other shade tolerant and water-seeking botanicals such as black cohosh (page 141) and blue flag iris (page 150).

HARVESTING THIS HERBAL ALLY

Parts Used: Woody rhizome, leaves, flowering tops

When to Harvest for Medicinal Potency: Harvest leaves and flowering tops as the flowers start to emerge under a waxing moon. Harvest rhizomes during late summer or early fall, also under a waning moon.

HERBAL REMEDY TIP

Lady's mantle is very effective when utilized as a tincture, tea, decoction, infusion, cream/salve or bath to soothe and protect. For a soothing tincture to ease dysregulated menstruation with a sense of boggy heat and stagnation, I suggest a tincture using two parts lady's mantle to one part black cohosh (page 24).

Peony (White or Red)

Paeonia lactiflora

Herbal Energetics: Cool/dry
Signatures: Sensual, divine

Peony is widely regarded in both Western and Eastern herbal medicine for its affinity for the female reproductive system. Peony can relieve menstrual complaints such as cramping, fullness and clotting, while also alleviating menopausal issues like hot flashes and bone loss. Peony lowers blood pressure and is particularly effective in relieving chest tightness and overall inflammation that results from liver stagnation due to alcoholism and medication use. It also is thought to reduce excessive sweating and can help relieve a high fever.

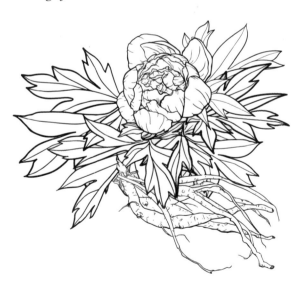

PLANT SNAPSHOT

Perennial
Zone: 3–8
Growth Habit: Mounding

GROWING THIS HEALING BOTANICAL

Light Requirements: Full sun to partial shade (protect from late afternoon rays in hotter regions)

Garden Placement: Peonies grow approximately 2 to 3 feet (0.6 to 0.9 m) tall and wide and are best planted as focal points near the midsection of a bed or border.

Soil Preference: Peonies like moderately rich, loamy, well-drained soils, but require frequent watering to keep the foliage lush and full throughout the season.

When to Plant: Peonies are best propagated by dividing the woody root system during mid-fall. Select and cut away large roots with feeder rootlets and at least three eyes and transplant them during a descending moon.

Best Growing Tips: Because peonies are not likely to bloom if planted deeply, bury roots more than 2 inches (5 cm) below the soil, and pull heavier mulch back from the crown before winter to prevent rot.

Garden Companions: Plant peonies with hydrangeas as they enjoy similar growing conditions.

HARVESTING THIS HERBAL ALLY

Parts Used: Woody roots

When to Harvest for Medicinal Potency: Dig up roots in the fall, cutting the side roots away from the crown, leaving at least two-thirds of the crown intact during a waning moon.

HERBAL REMEDY TIP

Craft a decoction of peony (page 23) and then infuse the resulting decoction with rose and chamomile as it cools. Sip as an iced tea to relieve a tendency toward hot flashes and excessive sweating.

Elecampane

Inula helenium

Herbal Energetics: Warm/dry
Signatures: Towering, radiant

Elecampane has an undeniable resinous flavor that is profoundly stimulating. Elecampane is specifically suggested by herbalists for thick, heavy mucus and an unproductive cough. It breaks up congestion in the sinuses and promotes drainage to restore respiratory health. This herb is ideal for those who experience nausea due to nasal drainage dripping into the digestive system. It can also stimulate delayed menses.

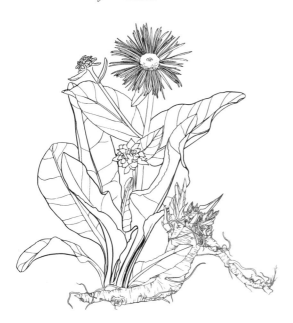

PLANT SNAPSHOT

Perennial
Zone: 3–9
Growth Habit: Tall, upright

GROWING THIS HEALING BOTANICAL

Light Requirements: Full sun to light shade

Garden Placement: As elecampane can grow quite tall, plant near the back of a bed or border.

Soil Preference: This botanical prefers moderately rich, loamy or silty, moisture-retentive soils.

When to Plant: Divide existing clumps of elecampane in fall by digging and selecting a rhizome at least 2 inches (5 cm) in length with an existing eye to transplant during a waning moon.

Best Growing Tips: Certain species of elecampane can grow upwards of 6 feet (1.8 m) tall, so choose your selection wisely to accommodate your space without overwhelming it.

Garden Companions: Elecampane is a great choice to pair with gravel root or boneset.

HARVESTING THIS HERBAL ALLY

Parts Used: Roots

When to Harvest for Medicinal Potency: Dig and divide elecampane roots near during a descending moon near the middle of fall once the foliage has mostly died back.

HERBAL REMEDY TIP

This resinous and bitter herb is most easily tolerated as a tincture (page 24). When dosing a child with this herb, I usually recommend mixing a dropperful of the tincture with a teaspoon of raw honey to make the experience more pleasant.

Fir

Abies species

Herbal Energetics: Cool/dry
Signatures: Towering, majestic

The sweet forest scent of fir is not only clarifying for the mind but offers great benefits for the respiratory system. Fir soothes and softens a stiff barking cough and respiratory congestion. A slow walk through a fir forest is thought to soothe asthma symptoms. This botanical is also an excellent antioxidant and is a wonderful cold and flu preventative when taken after exposure to viruses.

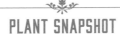

PLANT SNAPSHOT

Tree
Zone: 3–8
Growth Habit: Tall, straight, upright

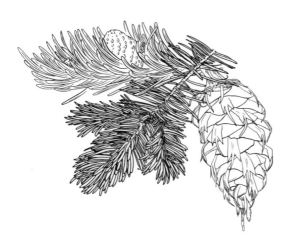

GROWING THIS HEALING BOTANICAL

Light Requirements: Full sun to partial shade

Garden Placement: Place fir trees where they will ultimately grow to their full-size potential—some species can grow well over 100 feet (30 m) tall.

Soil Preference: Firs like slightly acidic, humus-rich, moisture-retentive soils.

When to Plant: Firs are one of the few evergreens that are more easily propagated via cuttings (rather than waiting for seeds to germinate). Strip an 8- to 10-inch (20- to 25-cm) limb of auxiliary branches and needles on the lower two-thirds of the limb. Dip the cut edge in rooting hormone and plant 2 to 3 inches (5 to 7.5 cm) deep in moist potting medium during a waning moon.

Best Growing Tips: It is vitally important that firs are not harvested until they are well established and have been in the ground for at least 3 years to avoid stunting the growth of your tree.

Garden Companions: Underplant fir trees with violets and wild ginger.

HARVESTING THIS HERBAL ALLY

Parts Used: Needles

When to Harvest for Medicinal Potency: Harvest bright green growing tips in early spring during an ascending moon.

HERBAL REMEDY TIP

Breathe easy after sipping an infusion of fir needle (page 22) with a slice of orange and a cinnamon stick.

Horseradish

Armoracia rusticana

Herbal Energetics: Warm/dry
Signatures: Bold, assertive, aggressive

Quite possibly the most pungent herb of the apothecary, horseradish is a highly stimulating herb ideal for cold, damp conditions—this is an herb that gets things MOVING. Horseradish has a great affinity for the upper respiratory system, thinning mucus and opening the sinuses. This herb can bring a low, clammy fever to a head, while also warming joints and addressing chilblains. Horseradish is also highly diuretic and will promote full bladder elimination.

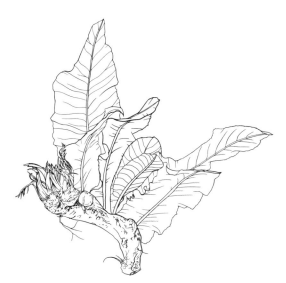

PLANT SNAPSHOT

Perennial
Zone: 3–9
Growth Habit: Deep roots with large clumping leaves

GROWING THIS HEALING BOTANICAL

Light Requirements: Full sun to partial shade (full sun is needed for peak pungency)

Garden Placement: Plant horseradish where it can remain relatively undisturbed for at least a year and near the middle to back of a bed or border due to their impressively sized leaves.

Soil Preference: Horseradish grows best in moist, moderately fertile loam.

When to Plant: Horseradish is most easily propagated by removing "sets" (smaller side roots of the larger main root) and transplanting during a waning moon.

Best Growing Tips: Note that once you plant horseradish, it is very likely to return year after year, even after a seemingly thorough harvest.

Garden Companions: Horseradish is a natural fungicide and may be helpful to grow next to plants prone to mold and mildew.

HARVESTING THIS HERBAL ALLY

Parts Used: Roots

When to Harvest for Medicinal Potency: Dig up horseradish roots in mid-fall during a waning moon.

HERBAL REMEDY TIP

Create a simplified fire cider by infusing 1 cup (240 g) of grated horseradish in 2 cups (480 ml) of raw apple cider vinegar. Strain after 2 months and sweeten the infusion with honey to taste. Take by the spoonful when the first sign of congestion hits.

Lungwort

Pulmonaria officinalis

Herbal Energetics: Cool/moist
Signatures: Soothing, grounded

For centuries, lungwort has been prized for its benefits for the respiratory system. Lungwort has slight moistening qualities that act to heal and protect lung tissues that are inflamed and damaged by prolonged respiratory illness. Its healing benefits extend similarly to the digestive system, helping to repair irritated tissues such as ulcers, fissures, and hemorrhoids. Lungwort is also a gentle diuretic, aiding the kidneys and bladder of complaints of stones and infection.

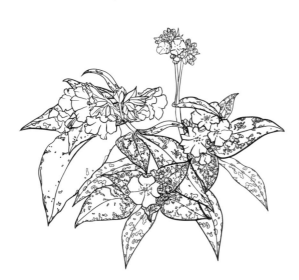

PLANT SNAPSHOT

Perennial
Zone: 5–8
Growth Habit: Clumping with flower spikes

GROWING THIS HEALING BOTANICAL

Light Requirements: Partial to full shade

Garden Placement: Plant lungwort en masse in a shady area to enjoy their early spring flowers and the lovely spotted foliage that persist until frost.

Soil Preference: Lungwort prefers moderate to rich, loamy, moist soils.

When to Plant: Most modern lungwort cultivars are hybridized and will only propagate "true" by division. Dig up plants in early fall and gently break them apart, transplanting during a waning moon.

Best Growing Tips: Lungwort needs evenly and consistently moist soils and should be planted where they receive shade and shelter but away from more aggressively thirsty plants or trees such as cottonwood.

Garden Companions: Plant lungwort with sweet woodruff to carpet a shady area with medicinal plants.

HARVESTING THIS HERBAL ALLY

Parts Used: Leaves

When to Harvest for Medicinal Potency: Gather leaves in spring and early summer during an ascending moon.

HERBAL REMEDY TIP

The healing mucilage benefits of lungwort are best experienced when sipped as a tea (page 22). Pair with spearmint for lung complaints and marshmallow for stomach and urinary tract irritation.

Wild Cherry (Chokecherry)

Prunus serotina, virginiana

Herbal Energetics: Cool/dry
Signatures: Guarding, protective

Wild cherry is an outstanding respiratory sedative for those with a painful, hacking, out-of-control cough. It calms erratic and fitful breathing while soothing greatly inflamed and infected tissue so that the person suffering can find rest, thereby allowing the body to heal the affected tissues. Note that due to the suppressive nature of this herb, it should not be used for those with diminished repository dysfunction such as prolonged pneumonia. Additionally, wild cherry can calm a cramping and aggressively upset stomach.

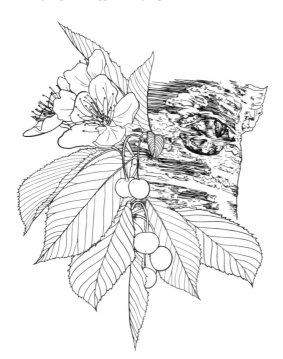

PLANT SNAPSHOT

Tree (serotina) or shrub (virginiana)
Zone: 2–8
Growth Habit: Erect, upright (serotina), large shrub (virginiana)

GROWING THIS HEALING BOTANICAL

Light Requirements: Full sun to partial shade

Garden Placement: Wild cherry should be grown where it has plenty of room to reach its full-size potential but can flourish in the open understory of larger trees.

Soil Preference: Wild cherry prefers moderately rich, moisture-retentive soils.

When to Plant: Wild cherry is most easily propagated by taking a limb cutting of 6 to 8 inches (15 to 20 cm) and dipping the cut end in rooting hormone and planting it in a sterile potting mix during a descending moon. Transplant to its final location once the roots are well established, also during a waxing moon.

Best Growing Tips: Due to its somewhat shallow root system, take care to properly plan placement as transplanting is not well tolerated.

Garden Companions: Underplant wild cherries with comfrey to nourish shallow roots of wild cherry.

HARVESTING THIS HERBAL ALLY

Parts Used: Bark, fruits (edible)

When to Harvest for Medicinal Potency: Gather bark from fallen or damaged limbs, or from cut trees or shrubs during an ascending moon.

HERBAL REMEDY TIP

Wild cherry bark makes an outstanding syrup (page 25) when first decocting with water until the liquid is reduced by half, then combining with cherry juice before completing the syrup.

Blue Flag Iris

Iris versicolor

Herbal Energetics: Cool/dry
Signatures: Bold, bright

Blue flag iris is highly regarded for its ability to clear the skin of troublesome acne and cystic breakouts. Blue flag iris tones the skin and reduces redness and inflammation. Internally, this botanical aids the liver in the body's natural detoxification process, which can greatly reduce cystic and hormonal acne. It also aids in the digestion of fats and promotes bladder and bowel elimination.

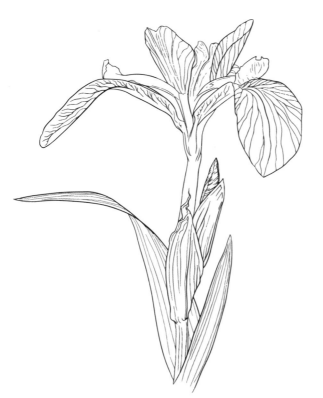

PLANT SNAPSHOT

Perennial
Zone: 2–7
Growth Habit: Clumping, strappy leaves with upright flower spikes

GROWING THIS HEALING BOTANICAL

Light Requirements: Full sun to partial shade

Garden Placement: Blue flag iris is a perfect choice for damp, even boggy soils near waterways.

Soil Preference: This botanical prefers moderately rich, moisture-retentive soils.

When to Plant: Divide rhizome clumps after flowering in mid-spring and transplant the lifted rhizomes to prepared soil during a descending moon.

Best Growing Tips: Blue flag irises will grow where other botanicals suffer—line the sides of an unsightly damp ditch where it can flourish and stabilize the slope.

Garden Companions: Grow blue flag iris with black cohosh, cottonwoods and birch.

HARVESTING THIS HERBAL ALLY

Parts Used: Rhizome

When to Harvest for Medicinal Potency: Lift rhizomes after they flower in mid- to late summer during a waning moon. Slice and dry immediately (fresh juices are a skin and mucous membrane irritant).

HERBAL REMEDY TIP

Tincture dried blue flag iris rhizome (page 24) and use during times of deep, painful cystic breakouts until skin clears and redness subsides.

Boneset

Eupatorium perfoliatum

Herbal Energetics: Cool/dry
Signatures: Beckoning

A somewhat confusing trick of etymology (and why we should not take common names at modern face value), boneset is not necessarily an herb for mending the skeleton. Instead, boneset received its moniker by its ability to relieve the overwhelming bone pain that is a symptom of what we now call dengue fever. As such, the boneset is an excellent remedy for viruses that include complaints of deep muscle and joint/bone ache and a hot, red-skinned fever. This potent antiviral herb also aids the digestive system, acting as a bitter that stimulates bile flow and enzymatic activity in the stomach.

PLANT SNAPSHOT

Perennial
Zone: 3–8
Growth Habit: Tall, upright

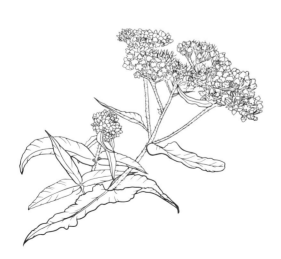

GROWING THIS HEALING BOTANICAL

Light Requirements: Full sun to partial shade

Garden Placement: Boneset thrives in wetland and heavy clay soil environments, making this herb ideal for naturalizing in hard-to-care-for damp, marshy meadows.

Soil Preference: This botanical thrives in moderately fertile, moist soils.

When to Plant: Sow boneset seeds in fall to allow for cold stratification but note that seed germination is somewhat sporadic and unreliable. Boneset is more easily propagated by root division. Dig up and separate clumps in mid-fall and transplant them during a waning moon.

Best Growing Tips: While boneset like fertile soils, it tends to become weak and floppy due to rapid growth when over fertilized. Top dress with compost rather than fertilizer to ensure a sturdier plant.

Garden Companions: Boneset develops a thick network of rhizomes and may choke out nearby plants. However, elecampane and gravel root (joe pye weed) are well suited to thrive in boneset's favored conditions.

HARVESTING THIS HERBAL ALLY

Parts Used: Leaves, flowers

When to Harvest for Medicinal Potency: Gather leaves and flowers during the growing season under an ascending moon.

HERBAL REMEDY TIP

To break an especially hot, agitated fever with extreme body ache, brew a strong infusion and sip until the fever breaks. Sweeten with honey to taste to offset the bitter flavor.

Bugleweed

Ajuga reptans

Herbal Energetics: Cool/dry
Signatures: Blanketing, robing

Bugleweed is known foremost as a styptic herb, capable of arresting bleeding from superficial wounds. It is also useful for any weepy complaints of the skin such as oily acne, oozy sunburn, oily scalp and cradle cap. A gargle of this herb is helpful for mouth sores and painful, bleeding gums. Historically, this botanical was also used for kidney and liver complaints, but modern herbalists shy away from internal use due to bugleweed's slight narcotic effect and potential for toxicity.

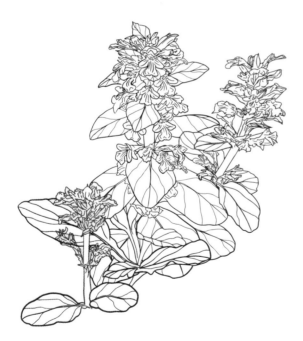

PLANT SNAPSHOT

Perennial
Zone: 3–9
Growth Habit: Creeping, mat-like

GROWING THIS HEALING BOTANICAL

Light Requirements: Full sun to partial shade

Garden Placement: Replace turf grass with bugleweed in areas that are relatively shady and prone to patchiness.

Soil Preference: Bugleweed prefers moderately fertile, moisture-retentive soils.

When to Plant: Divide existing clumps in late spring or early fall and transplant new clumps during a descending moon.

Best Growing Tips: Bugleweed grows quite densely and will outcompete grass and other small plants in its vicinity.

Garden Companions: Bugleweed is one of the few plants tolerant of juglone, so plant freely under black walnuts.

HARVESTING THIS HERBAL ALLY

Parts Used: Leaves, flowers

When to Harvest for Medicinal Potency: Gather leaves and flowers while in bloom during an ascending moon.

HERBAL REMEDY TIP

Tincture fresh bugleweed (page 24) with mint (page 41) and dilute in water for a daily gargle to address sore, red and bloody gums.

Therapuetic Actions Index

Agrimony: Anti-inflammatory, astringent, cholagogue, diuretic, hepatic, hypoglycemic, renal, styptic, vulnerary

Aloe: Anticancer, anti-inflammatory, anti-fungal, demulcent, diuretic, emollient, gastro-protective, immune-modulating, vulnerary

Amaranth: Anti-inflammatory, antioxidant, cardiovascular, diuretic, hypolipidemic, hypotensive, laxative, nutritive, styptic

Angelica: Analgesic, antibacterial, anticancer, antifungal, anti-inflammatory, antiseptic, antispasmodic, antiviral, astringent, cardiovascular, carminative, decongestant, diaphoretic, emmenagogue, expectorant, nervine

Arnica: Analgesic, anti-arthritic, anti-hematoma, anti-inflammatory, anti-microbial, antirheumatic, antitraumatic (physical or emotional), immune stimulating

Artichoke: Anti-inflammatory, antilipidemic, antioxidant, astringent, cardiovascular, digestive, diuretic, hypoglycemic, hypotensive, hepatic, laxative-metabolic, nutritive

Ashwagandha: Adaptogenic, aphrodisiac, anti-anemic, anti-inflammatory, anti-tumor, cognitive, immune-modulating neuro-protective, nervine, sedative (mild)

Astragalus: Antibacterial, anti-inflammatory, cardiovascular, hepatic, hypoglycemic, hypotensive, diuretic, (mild) immune stimulating, tonic

Bacopa: Antimicrobial, antioxidant, cardio-vascular, cognitive, digestive, hepatic, nervine, neuro-protective, nootropic

Bay: Antimicrobial, antiseptic, antispasmodic, carminative, diaphoretic, digestive, expectorant, tonic

Bee Balm: Antibacterial, antifungal, antioxidant, antiseptic, antispasmodic, antiviral, carminative, decongestant, diaphoretic, diffusive, emmenagogue, nervine, relaxant, stimulant

Beth Root: Anti-inflammatory, antispasmodic, astringent, emmenagogue, expectorant, styptic

Birch: Alterative, analgesic, anti-arthritic, antimicrobial, anti-inflammatory, antirheumatic, antiseptic, antispasmodic, astringent, diaphoretic, diuretic, expectorant, immune stimulating

Black Cohosh: Analgesic, anti-inflammatory, antirheumatic, antispasmodic, astringent, cardio-vascular, emmenagogue, nervine

Black Walnut: Antibacterial, antifungal, anti-inflammatory, antioxidant, antiparasitic, astringent, cardiovascular, digestive, nutritive

Blue Flag Iris: Anti-inflammatory, antibacterial, astringent

Boneset: Analgesic, antibacterial, anti-inflammatory, antiviral, diaphoretic, digestive, emetic, expectorant, nervine

Borage: Adaptogenic, anti-inflammatory, demulcent, expectorant, febrifuge, expectorant, galactagogue, nervine

Bugleweed: Astringent, antispasmodic, cardiac, emmenagogue, hypothyroid, nervine, sedative, vulnerary

Calendula: Anti-inflammatory, antimicrobial, antispasmodic, astringent, demulcent, emmenagogue, hemostatic, lymphatic, vulnerary

California Poppy: Analgesic, anti-inflammatory, antispasmodic, anxiolytic, nervine, sedative

Camellia: Antibacterial, anti-inflammatory, antilipidemic, antioxidant, antiviral, astringent, cardiac, cardio-vascular, neuroprotective, stimulant

Catmint: Anti-inflammatory, anti-microbial, antispasmodic, antitussive, astringent, carminative, diaphoretic, digestive, emmenagogue, expectorant, nervine, sedative

Cayenne: Analgesic, anti-arthritic, anti-inflammatory, antimicrobial, antioxidant, antirheumatic, antiseptic, antispasmodic, cardiac, cardiovascular, carminative, diaphoretic, decongestant, digestive, meta-bolic, nutritive, rubefacient, sialagogue

Chamomile: Alterative, analgesic, anti-inflammatory, antimicrobial, antihistamine, antioxidant, antispasmodic, astringent, cardiac, carminative, digestive, diuretic, emmenagogue, expectorant, hypoglycemic, hypotensive, nervine, nutritive, insect repellent, prostatic, sedative, vulnerary

Chaste Tree/Vitex: Analgesic, anti-androgen, anticancer, anti-inflammatory, antioxidant, antispasmodic, carminative, digestive, diuretic, emmenagogue, fertility, galactagogue, prostatic

Chickweed: Analgesic, alterative, anti-cell proliferate, antioxidant, antimicrobial, antihistamine, anti-inflammatory, antiseptic, demulcent, diuretic, hepatic, hypoglycemic, metabolic, nutritive, renal

Chicory: Alterative, anti-inflammatory, astringent, cholagogue digestive, diuretic, hepatic, hypoglycemic, laxative, metabolic

Chives: Anticancer, antioxidant, anti-microbial, cardiovascular, carminative, cognitive, digestive, hypotensive, immune stimulant, nutritive

Coltsfoot: Alterative, antitussive, demul-cent, diuretic, expectorant, vulnerary

Comfrey: Antibacterial, anti-hematoma, anti-inflammatory, anti-ulcerative, cell proliferate, vulnerary

Coriander: Analgesic, antimicrobial, antioxidant, antispasmodic, carminative, digestive, diuretic, hypoglycemic, hypotensive, renal

Cornflower: Anti-inflammatory, astringent, digestive, diuretic, hepatic, immune stimulant, vulnerary

Cornsilk: Antibacterial, anti-inflammatory, antispasmodic, astringent, diuretic, hepatic, hypotensive, prostatic, renal

Corydalis: Analgesic, antibacterial, anti-cancer, antifungal, anti-ulcerative, cardiac, cardiovascular, digestive, hepatic, sedative

Cottonwood: Analgesic, anti-cell proliferate, anti-inflammatory, antioxidant, antimicrobial, astringent, diaphoretic, expectorant, immune-modulating

Crampbark: Anti-inflammatory, antioxidant, antispasmodic, astringent, diuretic, emmenagogue, hypotensive, nervine, sedative (mild), tonic

Cranberry: Antibacterial, anticancer, antioxidant, astringent, diuretic, hepatic, hypoglycemic, nutritive

Dill: Anti-inflammatory, antispasmodic, carminative, digestive, galactagogue

Echinacea: Alterative, anti-inflammatory, antimicrobial, expectorant, immune-modulating, sialagogue, vulnerary

Elder: Antimicrobial, antioxidant, antirheumatics, antispasmodic, diaphoretic, diuretic, expectorant, immune-modulating, laxative

Elecampane: Anti-inflammatory, antispasmodic, antitussive, carminative, digestive, expectorant, nervine

Evening Primrose: Antidepressant, anti-inflammatory, antispasmodic, astringent, diuretic, emmenagogue, emollient (seed oil), nervine, sedative (mild), vulnerary

Eyebright: Antihistamine, anti-inflammatory, astringent, vulnerary

False Unicorn: Anti-abortifacient, anti-emetic, digestive, diuretic, emmenagogue, renal, uterine tonic

Fennel: Anti-inflammatory, antispasmodic, carminative, digestive, galactagogue, hepatic

Feverfew: Antibacterial, anti-inflammatory, astringent, diaphoretic, emmenagogue, hepatic, vasodilator

Fir: Anti-inflammatory, antiseptic, expectorant, respiratory, sedative

Garlic: Alterative, antilipidemic, antimicrobial, antispasmodic, cardiovascular, carminative, cholagogue, diaphoretic, expectorant, hypotensive, nutrient, stimulant, tonic, vulnerary

Gentian: Anti-acne, antimicrobial, anthelmintic, astringent, cholagogue, emmenagogue, hepatic, sialagogue

Gingko: Anti-inflammatory, cognitive, digestive, nervine, stimulant

Ginseng: Adaptogen, hypoglycemic, immune-modulating, stimulant, tonic

Goldenseal: Alterative, anti-inflammatory, antimicrobial, cholagogue, digestive, emmenagogue, expectorant, hepatic, laxative

Gravel Root: Anti-inflammatory, antilithic, antirheumatic, diuretic, renal

Ground Elder: Antirheumatic, diuretic, renal

Hawthorn: Anti-inflammatory, antioxidant, astringent, cardiovascular, hyotenisive

Helichrysum: Antihistamine, antimicrobial, antioxidant, antitussive, astringent, cholagogue, cicatriscant, diuretic, expectorant, hepatic, vulnerary

Holy Basil: Adaptogenic, analgesic, anti-arthritic, anticancer, anti-emetic, antihistamine, anti-inflammatory, antimicrobial, antimalarial, antioxidant antispasmodic, anthelmintic, astringent, cardiovascular, cognitive, hepatic, hypoglycemic, hypolipidemic, hypotensive, immuno-modulating, nervine, sedative

Honeysuckle: Analgesic, anti-inflammatory, antimicrobial, astringent, decongestant, diuretic, expectorant

Hops: Analgesic, antiseptic, antispasmodic, anxiolytic, astringent, diuretic, sedative

Horehound: Antispasmodic, astringent, cholagogue, digestive, emmenagogue, expectorant, vulnerary

Horseradish: Antimicrobial, antiseptic, carminative, decongestant, diffusive, expectorant, laxative, rubefacient, stimulating

Hydrangea: Anti-inflammatory, antilithic, diuretic, emmenagogue, renal

Hyssop: Anti-inflammatory, antispasmodic, carminative, diaphoretic, digestive, expectorant, nervine

Jamaican Dogwood: Analgesic, antispasmodic, nervine

Jewelweed: Antihistamine, anti-inflammatory, astringent

Juniper: Anti-inflammatory, antimicrobial, antirheumatic, carminative, digestive, diuretic, renal, rubefacient

Lady's Mantle: Alterative, anti-aging, anti-inflammatory, antimicrobial, antioxidant, astringent, coagulant, diuretic, emmenagogue, hepatic, hypoglycemic, hypotensive, lithontriptic, pro-collagen, vasodilator, vulnerary

Lamb's Ear: Absorbent, anti-inflammatory, antibacterial, antiseptic, astringent, vulnerary

Lavender: Antidepressant, anti-inflammatory, antimicrobial, antiseptic, antispasmodic, anxiolytic, astringent, carminative, cholagogue, hepatic, hypnotic, insect repellent, nervine, sedative, vulnerary

Lemon Balm: Antidepressant, anti-inflammatory, antimicrobial, antispasmodic, carminative, diaphoretic, digestive, hepatic, nervine

Licorice: Anti-inflammatory, antispasmodic, anti-ulcer, demulcent, emollient, expectorant, hepatic, hypertensive, laxative

Linden: Antispasmodic, astringent, demulcent (flowers), diaphoretic, diuretic, hypotensive, sedative

Lovage: Anti-inflammatory, astringent, diffusive, carminative, digestive, diuretic (strong), emmenagogue, hepatic, renal, sialagogue

Lungwort: Anti-inflammatory, astringent, carminative, demulcent, digestive, emollient, expectorant, styptic, vulnerary

Marshmallow: Anti-inflammatory, anti-ulcer, demulcent, diuretic, emollient, expectorant, laxative (mild), vulnerary

Meadowsweet: Analgesic, antacid, anti-emetic, anti-inflammatory, antimicrobial, antirheumatic, anti-ulcerogenic, astringent, carminative, diaphoretic, diuretic, febrifuge, immune-modulating, tonic

Mimosa: Antidepressant, nervine, sedative

Mint: Analgesic, anti-inflammatory, anti-emetic, antimicrobial, antispasmodic, carminative, diaphoretic, nervine

Motherwort: Antispasmodic, cardiovascular, emmenagogue, hepatic, hypotensive, nervine

Mugwort: Antidepressant, anti-inflammatory, antimicrobial, anthelmintic, astringent, carminative, cholagogue, digestive, hepatic, hypnotic, nervine

Mullein: Analgesic (flower), anti-inflammatory, antispasmodic, astringent (root), demulcent (leaf), expectorant, lymphatic, vulnerary

Mustard: Analgesic, anti-arthritic, anti-inflammatory, antimicrobial, carminative, decongestant (strong), digestive, diffusive, emetic, expectorant, stimulating

Navajo Tea: Alterative, analgesic, anthelmintic, anticancer, anti-inflammatory, antimicrobial, antioxidant, antispasmodic, antitussive, cholagogue, diuretic, hepatic, renal

Nigella: Anti-inflammatory, antioxidant, cardiovascular, carminative, cognitive, digestive, emmenagogue, galactagogue, hepatic, hypotensive, stimulant

Oak: Anti-inflammatory, antiseptic, astringent

Oats: Antidepressant, antispasmodic, anxiolytic, cardiovascular, demulcent, emollient, galactagogue, hypolipidemic, nervine, nutritive, trophorestorative, vulnerary

Oregano: Antimicrobial, antiseptic, antispasmodic, carminative, diaphoretic, diffusive, diuretic, expectorant, emmenagogue

Oregon Grape: Alterative, anti-inflammatory, antimicrobial, anti-emetic, cholagogue, expectorant, hepatic, tonic

Passionflower: Analgesic, antispasmodic, hypnotic, hypotensive, nervine

Peach: Anti-inflammatory, anti-emetic

Peony: Anticoagulant, anti-inflammatory, antispasmodic, astringent, diuretic, emmenagogue, nervine, sedative (mild)

Pine: Anti-inflammatory, antimicrobial, antioxidant, antispasmodic, decongestant, expectorant, nitritive, vulnerary

Pleurisy Root (Milkweed): Anti-inflammatory, antispasmodic, carminative, digestive, diaphoretic, expectorant

Pumpkin: Anthelmintic, anti-emetic, anti-inflammatory, antioxidant, diuretic, hypotensive, nutritive, pro-collagen, laxative, prostatic

Red Clover: Alterative, antioxidant, antispasmodic, diaphoretic, emmenagogue, nutritive

Red Raspberry: Astringent, emmenagogue, parturient, tonic

Rose: Anti-inflammatory, aphrodisiac, demulcent, emollient, vulnerary

Rosemary: Anti-inflammatory, antidepressant, antimicrobial, antispasmodic, astringent, carminative, cognitive, hypertensive, emmenagogue, rubefacient

Rue: Antimicrobial, antispasmodic, antitussive, cholagogue, emmenagogue, insecticidal

Sage: Anti-inflammatory, antimicrobial, antispasmodic, carminative, diaphoretic, digestive, diffusive, emmenagogue

Sassafras: Alterative, analgesic, anticoagulant, anti-inflammatory, antirheumatic, carminative, diaphoretic, digestive, diuretic, emmenagogue, renal

Sea Buckthorn: Anticancer, anti-inflammatory, antimicrobial, antioxidant, cardiovascular, emollient (seed), hepatic, immune-stimulating, vulnerary

Sea Holly: Anti-inflammatory, diaphoretic, diffusive, diuretic, expectorant, emmenagogue, hepatic, lymphatic

Skullcap: Antispasmodic, anxiolytic, hypotensive, nervine

Snapdragon: Antimicrobial, antioxidant, astringent, diuretic, hepatic, insecticidal, vulnerary

Solomon's Seal: Analgesic, anti-arthritic, anti-inflammatory, antirheumatic, antispasmodic, cardiovascular, demulcent, diuretic, emollient, sedative, vulnerary

Spilanthes: Analgesic, anti-inflammatory, antimicrobial, immune stimulant, numbing, sialagogue, stimulating

St. John's Wort: Antidepressant, antimicrobial, anti-inflammatory, astringent, nervine, vulnerary

Stinging Nettle: Alterative, antihistamine, anti-inflammatory, astringent, diuretic, hypotensive, nutritive, renal, tonic

Sunflower: Anti-inflammatory, antimicrobial, antirheumatic, cardiovascular, diaphoretic, digestive, diuretic, nutritive

Sweet Alyssum: Anti-inflammatory, antimicrobial, antioxidant, astringent, diuretic (strong)

Sweet Annie: Anti-inflammatory, antimicrobial, antihistamine, antiparasitic, astringent, digestive, diuretic

Sweet Woodruff: Analgesic, anti-inflammatory, antimicrobial, antiparasitic, astringent, decongestant, diuretic, vulnerary

Thyme: Antimicrobial, antispasmodic, anthelmintic, astringent, carminative, decongestant, diaphoretic, expectorant

Uva Ursi: Anti-inflammatory, antimicrobial, antiseptic, astringent, diuretic

Valerian: Antispasmodic, carminative, emmenagogue, hypnotic, hypotensive, nervine, sedative

Vervain: Antispasmodic, diaphoretic, galactagogue, hepatic, hypotensive, nervine, sedative, tonic

Violet: Alterative, anti-inflammatory, antioxidant, demulcent, diuretic, emollient, expectorant, nutritive

Wild Carrot: Antilithic, antirheumatic, antispasmodic, carminative, contraceptive, digestive, diuretic, emmenagogue

Wild Cherry: Anti-inflammatory, antispasmodic, antitussive, astringent, expectorant (relaxing), nervine

Wild Ginger: Analgesic, anti-inflammatory, diaphoretic, diuretic, emmenagogue, expectorant

Wormwood: Antidepressant, antimicrobial, anthelmintic, carminative, cholagogue, digestive, diuretic

Yarrow: Anti-inflammatory, astringent, antispasmodic, antimicrobial, diaphoretic, diuretic, emmenagogue, febrifuge, hepatic, hypotensive, styptic, vulnerary

Yucca: Analgesic, anti-arthritic, anti-inflammatory, antimicrobial, astringent, carminative, diuretic, laxative, vulnerary

Acknowledgments

Thank you to the Page Street team for honoring me with yet another opportunity to explore the world of herbalism with my readers. And to all my readers that have supported me through the years—I am so glad you joined me on this path.

Endless gratitude to my illustrator, tattoo artist and dear friend, Hanna Martin. Collaborating with you is every bit the joy that our friendship is. I am delighted to carry your art out into the world, not only on my skin, but with this book!

To every gardener that has inspired my passion for plants along the way, you have my endless appreciation. You are too numerous to mention and so many of you I will never meet. The world of plants seen through the lens of individual gardeners in parks, private and home gardens never ceases to inspire me to cultivate beauty in my own landscape.

To my fellow herbalists and garden writers—I swell with gratitude. Betsy, Pam, Amy, Kris, Teri, Colleen, Stephanie, Dawn and Melissa—your support and advice has been nothing short of amazing.

To my friends that have supported me through the book writing process, I feel so unbelievably supported. Ivy, Heather, Justin, Lore and Jessica—you guys have no idea how much you helped keep my sanity intact!

To my parents, Susan and David, and my stepfather Art, as well as my sisters Melissa, Kaitlin, and Erin—thank you for the love, inspiration and support.

To Grandad, this book is dedicated to you and Grandma. You both created the gardener in me.

To my daughters, son-in-law, and brand new grandson—your love and encouragement has been endless. Thank you with all my love.

And finally, to an amazing person in my life that reminded me about the metaphorical act of planting a seed. You plant something small and seemingly inert. You care for it with anticipation. Then one day, a hard exterior cracks and something amazing grows from a simple act of hope. Thank you.

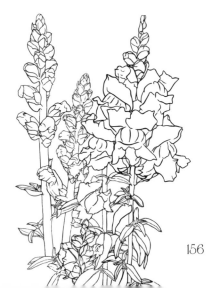

About the Herbalist

DEVON YOUNG is an herbalist, gardener, mother and writer living in the gorgeous and abundant Pacific Northwest. Devon is a graduate of the American College of Healthcare Sciences with a degree in Complementary and Alternative medicine but has spent a lifetime devoted to the study of plants. She can be found stalking garden centers and plant sales, locating the nearest botanical garden, taking innumerable plant photos and pulling over her truck to inspect the roadside flora. Devon will happily engage in riveting discussion of compost or the medicinal aspects of lichen with anyone that will join her for a cup of tea or a walk in the garden.

About the Illustrator

HANNA MARTIN lives with her family on beautiful Kalapuya land in the gorgeous Willamette Valley. She is a sought-after tattoo artist and co-owner of the women-owned A New Leaf Studio in the quaint little town of Monmouth, Oregon. Chlorophyll and creativity run through her DNA. The code Hanna lives by is to forever seek spiritual connection and knowledge through nature and art. Decades of gardening, a love of medicinal herbs and drawing in those quiet green spaces is where she finds solace.

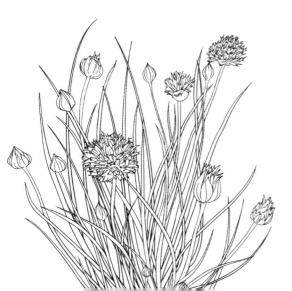

Index